The Living Needle

of related interest

Intuitive Acupuncture
John Hamwee
ISBN 978 1 84819 273 7
eISBN 978 0 85701 220 3

Developing Internal Energy for Effective Acupuncture Practice
Zhan Zhuang, Yi Qi Gong and the Art of Painless Needle Insertion
Ioannis Solos
ISBN 978 1 84819 183 9
eISBN 978 0 85701 144 2

The Spark in the Machine
How the Science of Acupuncture Explains the Mysteries of Western Medicine
Dr Daniel Keown MBChB, MCEM, LicAc
ISBN 978 1 84819 196 9
eISBN 978 0 85701 154 1

The Fundamentals of Acupuncture
Nigel Ching
Foreword by Charles Buck
ISBN 978 1 84819 313 0
eISBN 978 0 85701 266 1

The Compleat Acupuncturist
A Guide to Constitutional and Conditional Pulse Diagnosis
Peter Eckman MD, PhD, MAc (UK)
Foreword by William Morris
ISBN 978 1 84819 198 3
eISBN 978 0 85701 152 7

The Yellow Monkey Emperor's Classic of Chinese Medicine
Damo Mitchell and Spencer Hill
Artwork by Spencer Hill
ISBN 978 1 84819 286 7
eISBN 978 0 85701 233 3

The Luo Collaterals
A Handbook for Clinical Practice and Treating Emotions
and the Shen and the Six Healing Sounds
Dr David Twicken DOM, LAc
ISBN 978 1 84819 230 0
eISBN 978 0 85701 219 7

The Divergent Channels—Jing Bie
A Handbook for Clinical Practice and Five Shen Nei Dan Inner Meditation
Dr David Twicken DOM, LAc
ISBN 978 1 84819 189 1
eISBN 978 0 85701 150 3

THE LIVING
NEEDLE

Modern Acupuncture Technique

Justin Phillips

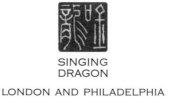

SINGING
DRAGON

LONDON AND PHILADELPHIA

First published in 2018
by Singing Dragon
an imprint of
Jessica Kingsley Publishers
73 Collier Street
London N1 9BE, UK
and
400 Market Street, Suite 400
Philadelphia, PA 19106, USA

www.singingdragon.com

Library of Congress Cataloging in Publication Data
A CIP catalog record for this book is available from the Library of Congress

British Library Cataloguing in Publication Data
A CIP catalogue record for this book is available from the British Library

ISBN 978 1 84819 381 9
eISBN 978 0 85701 339 2

Printed and bound in the United States

The accompanying videos can be downloaded from www.jkp.com/voucher using the code PHILLIPSNEEDLE.

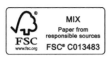

Contents

Online Video Content

The videos referred to throughout the text are available to download from www.jkp.com/voucher using the code PHILLIPSNEEDLE. The videos are referred to by number and demonstrate the following:

1. How to read needle sizes, the parts of a needle, how to remove it from packaging and how to insert and reinsert it into a guide tube

2. The needle grip and the principle of bracing fingers

3. Tubed insertion

4. Freehand insertion

5. Stretching

6. Pinching

7. Pressing

8. The three angles of insertion

9. Rotation

10. Lifting and thrusting

11. Plucking

12. Scraping

13. Shaking

14. Flying

15. Channel pressing

16. Needle pressing

17. Set the Mountain on Fire

18. Bring Heaven's Coolness

19. Midday, Midnight, Mortar-Pounding Pestle

20. Green Dragon Sways Its Tail

21. White Tiger Shakes Its Head

22. Green Turtle Burrows the Hole

23. Red Phoenix Flying

24. Surrounding Technique

INTRODUCTION

The practice of acupuncture is a conversation. It is a discussion between clinician and patient via mechanical stimulation. The needle, in and of itself, is not the treatment. Instead, it serves as a conduit: a translation device so that we, as physicians, can understand the occult language of another person's body and convey to that body the needed information for healing. This wondrous dialogue is initiated every time a needle enters the body, and is carried out with every lift, thrust, and rotation thereafter. To the skilled needle user, this is poetry—beautiful, intricate, and crafted with absolute purpose.

It is not necessary to have this relationship with the needle in order to practice acupuncture. In the thousands of years that acupuncture has been developed, many methods and approaches have come into being. I don't feel myself enough of a master to declare any approach better than another, though the skills we will discuss and describe in this book can expand any practice through their application.

The goal of this text is not to provide an in-depth description of specific "special" techniques, with their various perplexing names and complex applications, though some will be included, but instead, to offer a clear insight into the fundamental principles of needle technique, and why it can have a profound effect in the practice of Chinese Medicine.

The text will be organized generally around the flow of an actual patient encounter. We will begin with the basics of needle selection, move through patient and practitioner position, follow the insertion, proceed through the various mechanical actions we can take upon an inserted needle, and eventually finish with the withdrawal. Before beginning that journey together, I think it is important for you to understand my own personal philosophy of needling.

To me, the needle is not a static creature. It is not inserted and then left in place with a single manipulation to set its tone. Acupuncture is like tuning a piano. Hammers, mutes, and temperament strips are the tools of the tuner, and likewise pulse, tongue, and channel palpation are the diagnostic methods we use to see if the human instrument is in tune. The needle is the wrench with which we adjust out-of-tune strings. A piano tuner does not play a chord once, twist the wrench, and then move on. To the contrary, it is a constant interplay between sounding and adjusting, and at times the initial adjustments might change. A string that was tightened a moment before might now be loosened or further tightened in relation to another string's adjustment.

Acupuncture is like this.

One of the greatest attributes of Traditional Chinese Medicine (TCM) is that its power exists in the moment. It is present in the room with the patient at that instant, and not only responds to the individual as they are, but also adapts with changes that occur in the course of a treatment. This is one of the reasons that TCM has so defied modern testing, which presupposes that something done once will necessarily be done the same way every time. From TCM theory we know this is not true, but that in each moment we change and adapt. More than any other tool of the TCM clinician, such as herbs, acupuncture gives us the opportunity to be completely present with our patients in those moments, and likewise, respond to them very much as *they* are. Additionally, we can be present very much as *we* are. In needle therapy, it is impossible to separate the provider from the treatment.

Because of this, everything in this book should serve only as a guide. In the end, the experiences of each individual practitioner are what will determine the final choices made in treatment, whether it is what needles to use, or what manipulations are necessary. I cannot tell you what it feels like for you to touch a needle, or for you to feel a patient's tissues respond. I can only tell you what I experience. Only through your own experimentation and constant practice will you be able to develop your personal vocabulary of acupuncture treatment. They say a good teacher does not show you the destination, but only points the way. In the case of needle therapy, it is impossible to do otherwise. This book will show a path, but it is up to you to walk it.

To truly become a skilled needle therapist is a process of thousands of hours, needle in hand and mind in the moment. So let us begin.

1: **THE NEEDLE**

The modern, or filiform needle, is the core of the practice of acupuncture; not of TCM, mind you, as a distinction must be drawn between needle therapy and the broader practice of Chinese Medicine. Nevertheless, in the case of acupuncture itself, the needle is the key tool. It is critical for the acupuncture clinician to be intimately familiar with these needles, and the different sizes, shapes, and brands that are available. Just like a painter must be familiar with the brushes of their craft, which will each be utilized to produce different kinds of brush strokes to create an image, so too must the needle therapist know their needles, particularly when and how to use them. Just like a painter, the clinician will also find their favorite tools among the many needles available.

The historical development of the modern acupuncture needle is a rich story; however, it is one that we will not be telling here. There are many histories written about this practice that more than adequately detail the evolution of our tools. Instead, we will focus on what the needles have become, and how to best understand what we will be facing when the time comes to select a needle for use in treatment.

PARTS OF THE NEEDLE

The modern needle is divided into five, or sometimes four parts, depending on the brand and the design of the needle. Each part has significant factors that are worth noting. Those parts are:

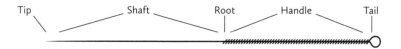

Tip

The tip of the needle is what will initially pierce the skin upon insertion. Because of this, the tip of the needle can significantly influence the sensation to the patient. There are two principal types when it comes to the tip of a needle. They are:

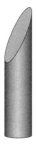

The bevel tip: This type of tip is not as common as it once was. The cut is simply angled across the line of the round needle body. This means that the needle has an inclination to pull across the plain of the bevel, rather than traveling straight. The leading edge is usually slightly broader, therefore tending to cut tissue rather than cleanly passing through. This is the type of tip that is found on most hypodermic needles. Not many brands still bevel tip their needles.

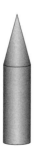

The center tip: This type of tip has become the standard for acupuncture needles. The center tip allows the needle to travel more cleanly into the body without unwanted shifting. It also causes less general tissue damage in its passage. The degree or precision will vary somewhat from brand to brand, as will the angle of the tip, but in general, all center tips will yield similar results.

Shaft

The shaft of the needle is a term for the portion between the tip and the handle. This is the part of the needle that, following the tip, will be inserted into the patient's body. For this reason, the shaft is very important when selecting needles for use, as your decision will directly impact the patient's sensations during treatment. One of the main factors in relation to the shaft is the size, which will be detailed in a later section. For the moment, what we will address is the smoothness.

There are two factors that will affect the smoothness of the needle. One is the quality of metal, which, by its nature, is porous. The pores will lead to a sense of roughness upon insertion and manipulation of the needle. The lower the grade of the metal, the more porous it is, and the rougher the shaft will be. This rough quality will cause the needle to "stick" and "grab" at tissue as it passes through the skin, or is rotated. The specific materials of acupuncture needles will be detailed in a later section.

The other factor that can dramatically influence the smoothness of the needle is whether it is coated or not. In recent history, it has become popular to coat acupuncture needles with silicone, or similar substances. Unlike metal, these coatings can be almost completely smooth, leading to much less sticking and grabbing of the tissue. This can be both good and bad. While the smoother needle will tend to lead to easier insertions (and therefore often less discomfort for the patient), it will also lead to a decrease in sensory input for the clinician, as the needle is less engaged with the surrounding tissue.

Neither needle should be considered superior to the other. It is entirely possible to insert an uncoated needle smoothly and without pain, just as it is possible to fully engage the tissue with a coated one. It is only important to understand the different natures of these two needles and the relevant advantages and disadvantages when making a needle selection. The only way to really understand what the treatment of the shaft means is for the practitioner to experiment with each and discover what works best for their own personal approach to needle work.

Root

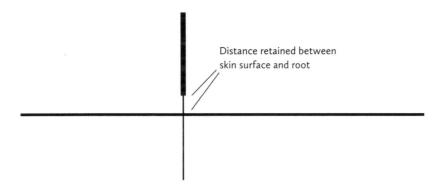

Distance retained between skin surface and root

The root is concurrently the least and most important part of the needle: least important in that it serves no purpose in the actual practice of needling, as it is simply where the shaft meets the handle; most important in that it is the point where a needle is most likely to break, though with modern needle technology it is unlikely that a needle will break. However, in the event that it does, the root becomes all important. When inserting an acupuncture needle, we should never insert the shaft all the way up to the root. Some small portion of the shaft should always be left extending beyond the surface of the skin so that, should the needle break, there will be a bit of shaft by which the needle might be grasped and removed from the tissue.

DO NOT INSERT A NEEDLE TO THE ROOT

It is important always to leave a portion of the needle extending beyond the skin before the root. This will prevent the needle from being lost in the skin should it break, an event that would require surgical intervention to remove the body of the needle. Should a needle break and a portion of it has been left exposed, the patient should be counseled not to move while the needle is removed with tweezers or hemostat.

Handle

The handle is the portion of the needle that is grasped by the practitioner. There are a wide variety of handles available today. Each has its own advantages, and practitioners are encouraged to try a wide variety to determine which is most conducive to their style of practice, or best suited for a specific situation.

There are a few obvious treatments that lend themselves to specific types of needle handles. For instance, if the provider is planning to perform e-stim treatment, a needle with a metal handle can be helpful. For a thin needle or shallow insertion, a plastic handle can be of benefit, as it is lighter and will pull on the needle less after insertion. For certain techniques, the wire-wound handle can assist by giving the clinician something to push or scratch against. There is no absolute in the selection of needle handles. It becomes a personal choice through experiment and experience.

Tail

The tail, or loop of the needle, like the root, has little significance in actual treatment processes. Many needles no longer have a tail. The original purpose of the tail had to do with the manufacturing of the needles themselves. Most needles were made of a single piece of wire which was bent over and wrapped around itself to create the handle. A sharp bend would make the wire more likely to break, so the wire would be bent into a large loop which could then be curved back around into the handle. With modern manufacturing techniques, the issue of breaking is significantly less, and many needle brands no longer include the loop on the end of the needle.

UNDERSTANDING NEEDLE SIZE

Over the years, needles have been sized many different ways. They have been described by gauge, both Chinese and Japanese (which count opposite directions), by inches, and by millimeters. At this point, most needle companies have settled on a standard of millimeters for conveying needle size, so that is the measurement we will use here. In reading needle sizes, there are two numbers that are relevant: thickness and length. The sizes are typically displayed somewhere on the needle packaging like this: thickness (mm) x length (mm).

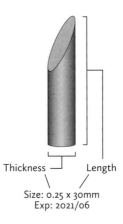

Thickness — Length

Size: 0.25 x 30mm
Exp: 2021/06

Thicknesses tend to range from .16 mm up to .30 mm, though both smaller and larger needles do exist. When considering the thickness of a needle, there are several factors that a clinician should take into account. First, a thicker needle will often elicit greater sensation from a patient. It can also create more effect in more delicate tissue—for instance, a thicker needle in the face is more likely to cause bruising. Conversely, a thinner needle will engage the tissue less, provide less sensation to the clinician, and be more difficult should a freehand insertion be desired.

The length of the needle is also measured in millimeters, though needles are often verbally described in cun measurements (traditional

Chinese measurement of a person's thumb width at the knuckle, the "Chinese inch"). This is the classical measurement method of needles, but as cun are not a standard size in all cases, millimeters have become the preferred method. There is a basic correlation between millimeters and cun, however, with 25 mm being generally agreed upon as the length of 1 cun. The length being described is the length of the shaft, not the full length of the needle.

A 1 cun needle will range anywhere from 25 mm to 30 mm. The reason for the range is that if a clinician desires a 1 cun depth of insertion and wants to avoid inserting to the root of the needle, the extra 5 mm is necessary.

In selecting needle length, the chief concern is the anatomy at the area of insertion. A shorter needle will be used where there is less tissue, or a possible risk of injury with deep insertion. A longer needle becomes necessary when working in thicker tissue, or where there is a need to move into deeper structures, such as joints and larger muscle groups. Needle length and depth can also be related to treatment principles, with more external disorders normally being treated at shallower depths, but that is a topic for a different book.

NEEDLE MATERIALS

Acupuncture needles have been made of a wide variety of materials over the years. Most needles today are made of high-grade surgical steel, as this is considered the safest, most durable, and most cost-effective material. A lower-quality needle will often have more nickel in its steel composition as a byproduct of inferior production methods. This can lead to stiffer and more brittle needles, and as nickel is one of the most common metal allergies, patients may manifest with skin reactions.

There are needles available in other materials as well, such as gold, silver, and copper. Various special properties are often attributed to these metals. Depending on the school, gold is considered to be the best for tonification, while silver is used to sedate; or alternatively, gold is tonifying, silver is neutral, and copper is sedating or cooling. These needles have become less popular as acupuncture has shifted to single use, disposable needles, and the cost of constantly replacing these needles has become prohibitive. In place of needles, some practitioners will use probes made of these metals, known in Japanese acupuncture practices as teishin, which do not pierce the skin, but are considered to create the appropriate stimulation through pressure and contact.

SELECTING A NEEDLE

All the factors we have covered should be taken into consideration when selecting an acupuncture needle for treatment. However, none of these factors mean anything without the hands-on experience to really understand the various attributes. The information in this chapter should act not as absolute gospel, but as signposts for what to look at and think about as different needles are used. A practitioner beginning to explore needling should endeavor to try as many different needles as possible. Only by determining what a clinician wants to accomplish, and understanding how these attributes of the needles affect a treatment, can that treatment and its outcome be effectively brought together **(see Video 1)**.

2: **INITIAL CONSIDERATIONS**

SAFETY CONCERNS

Before we begin to discuss the position of the patient or the posture of the provider, it is necessary to touch, at least briefly, on the primary safety concerns that might face the TCM clinician. Adverse effects are not common in the practice of Chinese Medicine and can be minimized by careful attention, but it is a mistake to imagine that they are impossible, and such thinking can lead to careless choices.

Pneumothorax

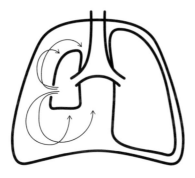

Pneumothorax occurs when damage to the lung tissue causes air to leak into the chest cavity, changing the internal pressure and causing the lung to collapse. This can occur in acupuncture if the needle touches the delicate tissue of the lung, causing a puncture or small tear.

Pneumothorax is very uncommon in the modern practice of acupuncture, especially with the increased training in anatomy at TCM schools. That being said, it remains the most common, severe complication of needle therapy. There are several points on the body where the possibility of touching the lungs with a needle exists, the most common being on the chest, back, and tops of the shoulders.

The needle making contact with a lung is not usually a result of insertion or manipulation, but rather poor consideration of the needle's possible movement during the duration of treatment. That is to say, a needle placed in an area of muscular contraction might move in or out if the patient shifts, or clothes which have been pulled aside can slide and shift during treatment, applying pressure to a needle. A careful practitioner can select needles of an appropriate size to limit risk of deep puncture around the lung, and utilize needle angle (discussed in a later chapter) to limit risk of a needle being pushed deeper and limiting total depth.

Even with the most careful practices, it is important to be aware of the basic signs and symptoms of pneumothorax. In most cases of acupuncture induced conditions, the onset will be gradual, and the primary signs will be shortness of breath and a persistent cough. If a patient presents with these issues and has had needles in an area where pneumothorax is a risk, they should be immediately referred to a hospital. This is without exception. While it is true that most cases of mild pneumothorax are self-resolving, it must always be considered an emergent condition.

Hematoma

Hematoma, or bruising, is the most common non-emergent side effect of needle therapy. The best way to deal with bruising is patient education. It is almost impossible to completely prevent bruising over the course of years of clinical practice. It is therefore wise to prepare your patients for the possibility. Acupuncture bruises are often painless and typically very small—about the size of a pencil eraser. Certain areas are more prone to significant bruising, such as the face, especially around the eyes, and these are areas where a clinician should take extra care and avoid excess needle movement.

If a patient experiences bruising, the best treatment is simply time. As the bruise is not dangerous in any way, it will resolve itself. If the patient does feel any soreness, or if they desire a faster resolution, topical substances such as arnica or other trauma reducers can be recommended.

Needle Shock

Needle shock occurs in 5–7 percent of acupuncture treatments. More correctly called vasovagal syncope, needle shock is a rapid drop in heart rate and blood pressure, driven by an adverse reaction in the central nervous system. Signs of needle shock are pallor, sudden sweating, dizziness, and nausea. In severe cases, the patient might have a brief loss of consciousness.

Syncope (fainting) can be caused by a number of triggers, and acupuncture is only one of them. People will often experience a vasovagal response at the sight of blood, a sudden shock, or even standing for too long. In the case of needle therapy, the response is usually a result of strong needling combined with a patient's nervousness about treatment. It can be aggravated if the patient hasn't eaten for some time before the treatment, as lower blood glucose levels have been shown to increase the chances of a vasovagal reaction. (Although poor hydration is not a risk factor for syncope, a dehydrated patient will often find needle insertion and manipulation more uncomfortable, therefore it is wise to also encourage drinking plenty of fluids before a treatment.)

If a patient begins to show the signs of possible needle shock, the needles should be removed immediately. The patient should be put in a comfortable position that minimizes the chance of falling should they lose consciousness. They can be given a sugary juice, such as orange juice, as an increase in blood glucose will generally help with the symptoms. Many clinicians will keep juice or sugar water on hand for just this purpose. In addition, moxa on St 36 (Zusanli), 3 cun below the lower border of the patella, can decrease the vasovagal response and reduce the needle shock symptoms.

The best treatment for needle shock is prevention. Advising patients to eat prior to treatment, creating a comfortable treatment environment, and educating the patient on what to expect during the treatment will significantly decrease the chance of an incident during treatment.

Stuck Needle

On occasion, a needle might get stuck in the patient's tissue. This is easily fixed and involves very little actual discomfort for the patient. In most cases, a stuck needle results from the tissue either winding around the needle because of rotation, or simply a spasm around the needle because of strong stimulation. If the issue is suspected to be winding, then the needle can be twisted the other way several times to release it. If the issue is spasm, or if rotation doesn't free the needle, the clinician can massage the tissue around the needle to cause it to relax and free the needle. If the needle remains stuck, a second needle can be inserted and lightly manipulated in proximity to the stuck needle, which will usually cause the first needle to become free. If the needle cannot be removed by any of the described methods, or if there is significant pain for the patient, it will be necessary to refer them out to have the needle surgically removed.

PATIENT POSITIONING

Once the initial work of intake, diagnosis, and treatment plan is completed, the patient must be positioned for needling. The two most common positions are face up and face down, or supine and prone. These are typically the most comfortable positions for patients to remain in for the duration of treatment. Patients might also be treated while lying on their side, while seated, and in some cases, even while standing. Patient positioning is a fairly straightforward process, but there are several factors that should be considered.

Safety is always first. This is to say that if a patient has compromised balance or impaired mobility, there might be restrictions on how they can be positioned. For instance, it would be unwise to place a patient with impaired balance in a standing position for treatment, or perhaps even seated. Another example would be a patient who is wheelchair-bound and cannot effectively climb up and down onto a treatment table, and therefore must be treated while seated. The practitioner must also remember that an acupuncture treatment often lasts 25–30 minutes, so the patient must be comfortably positioned for the duration of the treatment.

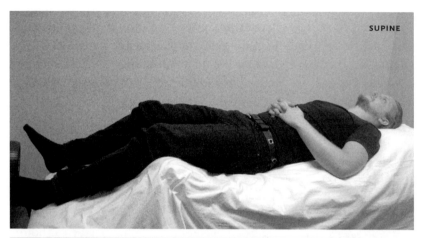

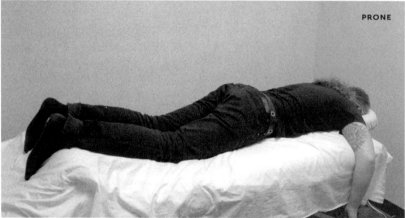

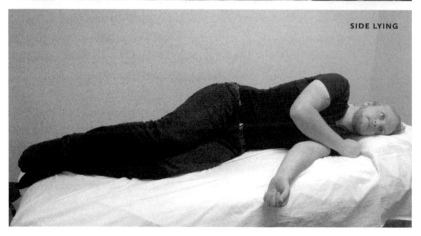

Second, the needs of treatment must be factored into position. If the practitioner wants to use points on the patient's back, it will be impossible for them to be in a supine position. If points on both the front and the back are necessary, either a side lying or seated position will be necessary.

Patient Comfort

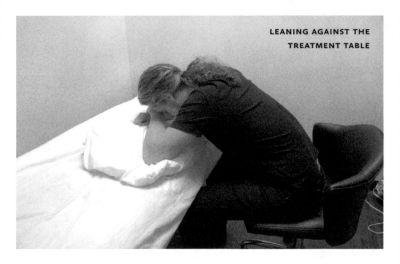

LEANING AGAINST THE
TREATMENT TABLE

It is worth noting that in more difficult positions, steps can be taken to maximize patient comfort. For instance, in a seated treatment the patient can lean against the treatment table or recline, and in a standing treatment they could be allowed to brace against the table or the wall to assist their balance.

The final consideration is the comfort of the practitioner themselves. The clinician will need to reach all the points to be treated, and the patient's position should ideally allow for this access to be natural and easy. If it is difficult for the provider to reach the patient, it will be hard for them to create the treatment process that they desire. Practitioner posture will be discussed in the next section.

It is important to note that in positioning a patient, I have put these considerations in the order of importance. The safety of the patient is always the provider's most central concern. After that, the needs of the patient should be considered, and then the needs of the provider. Optimally, all of these considerations can be addressed, but that is not always the case.

PATIENT COMMUNICATION

Although it is not always considered, good patient communication can have a profound impact on both patient comfort and safety. Many patients are unfamiliar with acupuncture treatments, but even those who have received therapy before may experience sensations that are outside the realm of their past exposure. Describing to your patient what to expect before a treatment, from typical sensations of needling to treatment duration, can lead to a better treatment experience. Often, patients will relate to their provider that they are experiencing pain during treatment, but they may simply be experiencing an unusual sensation for which they were not adequately prepared. A little bit of coaching can help a patient differentiate between normal sensations of needle therapy and pain, which will then help a clinician make well-grounded decisions in relation to adjustments.

Common sensations a patient might feel which are normal to acupuncture treatment are warmth, pressure, mild numbness or tingling, and even a very mild ache like a sore muscle. All of these are simply signs of the body's response to the needle and should not require any adjustment of the treatment protocol. If any of the sensations grow too strong or create actual pain or discomfort for the patient, adjustment or response might be required on the part of the clinician.

There are several negative sensations common to an acupuncture treatment that the clinician should bear in mind. A sharp, pinching pain similar to insertion, or even lingering after insertion, usually means the skin receptors are still being aggravated by the needle. Guiding the needle slightly deeper into the tissue will usually bring relief. A brief and localized burning sensation usually indicates contact with a dense area of capillaries and mild subcutaneous bleeding. This sensation will usually pass quickly, though if it is uncomfortable for the patient, the area can be lightly massaged, which will usually disperse the sensation. An electrical feeling, especially one that travels quickly to another part of the body, indicates proximity to a nerve. This sensation should not be pursued, and the needle is either withdrawn slightly or re-angled before continuing insertion. A very strong ache could indicate proximity to a major vessel, and like the nerve, should be avoided instead of pushed. Be it nerve or vessel, as both structures are typically thin and easily evaded, the point can still be treated by carefully adjusting the needle angle to move around them.

Explaining to a patient the process of the entire treatment, should they have an issue during therapy, can eliminate many problems before they arise. Patients are less likely to move around, adjust clothing, or leave the table if they have been informed of the risks. This also gives the patient a chance to voice any concerns or ask any questions prior to the beginning of treatment.

There is an additional benefit to this sort of patient counseling. Many people in our society are decidedly disconnected from their body and its physical sensations, and this may be your chance to offer a reconnection. How often is someone heard to say, "I haven't missed a day of work in 40 years?" This is said with pride, as if the ability to ignore the input of the body and its needs is a positive thing.

Another example is the patient who claims their system functions well—digestion, for example—but upon further questioning, it emerges there are many complications within that system. Perhaps the patient experiences gas, bloating, and acid reflux, but the symptoms are merely ignored. In such cases, engaging the patient in the physical sensations during needling can be a powerful step in reconnecting them to the signals of the body.

PROVIDER POSTURE

It would be impossible to overemphasize the importance of good posture for the provider, though we are not referring to what is considered "classically" good posture. A number of modern studies have suggested that what is commonly understood as good posture is not actually beneficial, and for the purpose of needling, is unimportant. In fact a number of "good" postures can be as much of an impediment to good needle work as bad posture. For instance, a martial horse stance (familiar to most as a position with feet spread and knees deeply bent), although considered to be excellent structural alignment, can prove excessively strenuous for a provider who hasn't trained to assume such positions. In the image below you can clearly see the increased weight the body must endure under poor posture.

Rather than "good" posture, I prefer to emphasize "natural" posture. This is a posture where the clinician feels comfortable and relaxed. The clinician should avoid excessive leaning or hunching, along with crouched or cramped positions that are difficult to assume, hard to hold, and challenging to move from afterward. Such positions put undue strain on the body, and leave a provider feeling unsteady. This sense of instability will be conveyed to the patient through the needle contact.

POSTURE AND WEIGHT DISTRIBUTION

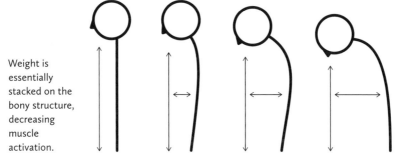

Weight is essentially stacked on the bony structure, decreasing muscle activation.

Increased hunching or leaning will increase the distance from skeletal alignment and the amount of muscular force needed to hold the shape.

More importantly, this body tension will make it profoundly more difficult to maintain the sensitivity and focus necessary for optimal needle work. The more tense a muscle, the less aware it is of subtle stimuli, the very information that is so critical to masterful treatment. The clinician should always attempt to create a stable position for themselves during each part of treatment: insertion, manipulation, and removal.

It is not necessary for the provider to possess legs of steel in order to create this alignment. In fact, with some planning, very little effort is usually necessary. Adequate space around a treatment table, a convenient stool, and correct table height are all important parts of engaging the patient from a comfortable position.

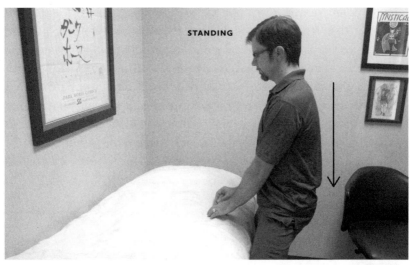

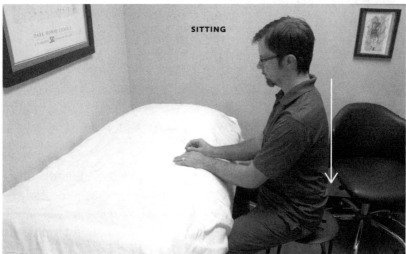

3: THE INSERTION

Once the points have been selected and both the patient and provider are in position, it is time to insert the needles. There are four primary concerns during insertion that will be discussed. First is the needle grip, second is the method of insertion, third is the depth of insertion, and fourth is the angle of insertion.

NEEDLE GRIP

Before it is possible to insert a needle, it is necessary to hold a needle. There are many ways to hold a needle, and though several will be illustrated here, the clinician must determine what grip is most comfortable for them. There are several standard ideas that must be considered in any needle grip. These are the three "Ss"—soft, secure, and stable.

First, the grip should be soft. Just like the provider's posture, a grip that is excessively tight or tense will detract from the sensitivity to the needle, and to the patient beyond it. In addition, a grip with excessive force will incline the provider to push and grind with the needle rather than to skillfully guide it.

Second, the grip should be secure. Although it is undesirable to over-grip the needle, it should also not be excessively loose in the fingers. Without positive connection to the handle, it is just as impossible to read the information coming from the needle as it would be with too tight a grip. Too loose a grip can lead to fumbling with the needle, which can both negatively impact the manipulation and create discomfort for the patient.

Last, the grip must be stable. A stable grip is not only a factor of how the needle is held, but how the hand is controlled in relationship

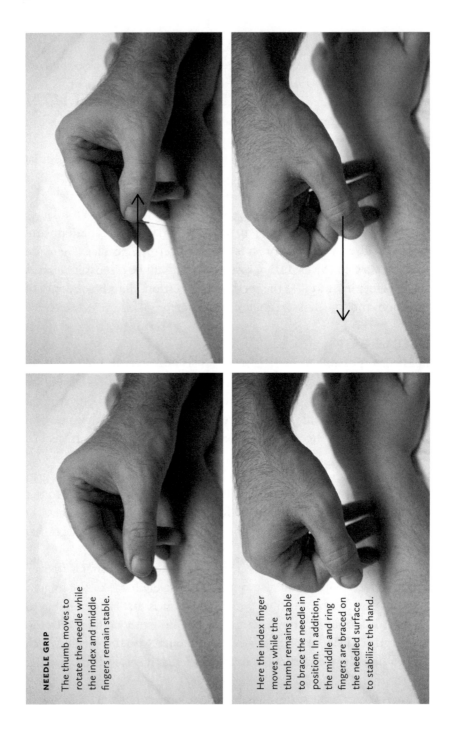

NEEDLE GRIP

The thumb moves to rotate the needle while the index and middle fingers remain stable.

Here the index finger moves while the thumb remains stable to brace the needle in position. In addition, the middle and ring fingers are braced on the needled surface to stabilize the hand.

to the patient. Fingers not in contact with the needle can be used to brace against the table, or the patient's body (which can also increase the connection between patient and practitioner), and the wrist can be braced with the other hand. The critical aspect of grip stability is that the practitioner should minimize any needle movement generated by either the hand or fingers, other than what is desired for treatment.

Another aspect of grip stability is the bracing finger. This means that in rotation or other dynamic movements, there is generally a moving finger, and a bracing finger that does not move. This non-moving finger will help limit excess needle movement beyond the desired stimulation **(see Video 2)**.

METHOD OF INSERTION

There are many ways that a needle can be inserted and many special methods that have been developed by clinicians over the years. However, for the purpose of clarity, we will be focusing on the broader concepts of insertion methods. There are two main areas of consideration in insertion methods: tube or freehand, and one- or two-handed.

Tube Insertion

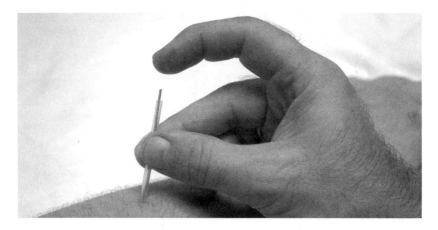

The guide tube, used in tube insertions, came into use in 17th-century Japan, when a blind acupuncturist named Waichi Sugiyama created it in order to insert thinner needles without causing pain. His schools received state recognition in Japan, leading to his methods becoming widespread, and today many acupuncturists use guide tubes. The guide tube allows for a very quick tapping insertion, while also limiting the possible depth of initial insertion, making tube insertions reliably safe.

In a tube insertion, the guide tube will be pressed to the skin at the selected point, or held slightly above it, and then the needle is tapped into the skin. When using a guide tube, it is important to secure the needle in the tube as it is brought to the skin. This is to prevent both the needle from falling out onto the floor, and any discomfort for the patient. The needle should be kept up in the body of the guide tube, and only allowed to move into contact with the skin once the guide tube is in place, when the practitioner is ready for actual needle insertion. If the needle drops to the mouth of the guide tube, or even below it, it will prick the patient's skin as it is moved into position.

Inserting a Needle into a Tube

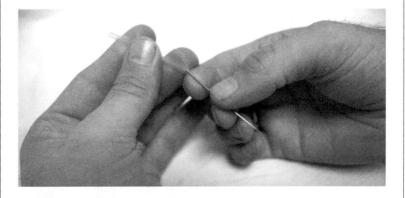

Some needles come with individual guide tubes; others will come with a pack of needles and a single guide tube. Regardless, it might at times be necessary to place a needle into a guide tube. When putting a needle into a tube, it is important to insert it handle first. This prevents accidental needle sticks in the event that the needle misses the tube (see Video 1).

Once the needle is in place, it should be inserted with a single strong tap of the finger. "Hesitation hurts" is an adage that should be kept in mind during needle insertion. The most sensitive part of the skin is the surface, so hesitant insertions that linger near the surface, or move in too slowly, are far more uncomfortable for a patient then a single, clean insertion. There are specific techniques where this is not the case—where a lighter insertion, or an insertion not to the full depth allowed by the guide tube is desired—but as a general rule, unless a specific goal is in mind, it is best to insert the needle fully in a single tap **(see Video 3)**.

Freehand Insertion

The other method of needle insertion is freehand. This is the insertion of a needle without the guide tube. In this method, the needle is held directly in the hand and inserted into the skin. This method is considered to be more difficult than tube insertions because the initial push through the skin must be accomplished unaided, and there is no tube to prevent the needle from bending. The key to successful freehand insertion is to move at the speed which the tissue will accept, and to make very small adjustments to the pressure being supplied to the needle. There is a tendency to initially push too hard, which will cause the needle to bend. Once the needle bends, the clinician will release almost all the pressure of the push, leading to not enough force to get through the skin. The reaction is to push harder to get through the skin, and the needle bends again. If, however, these adjustments are made more slowly and gradually, the happy medium, where the needle will insert into the skin, may be discovered.

In addition, a very light and quick back and forth rotation of the needle will help keep it from bending. The core lesson to bear in mind is that it is not necessary to insert a needle "fast" in order to avoid patient discomfort; rather, it is important to insert the needle smoothly, ideally in one continuous motion with even and consistent pressure. To accomplish this, it is important to focus on developing sensitivity and awareness of needle sensation. It is easy to look at the needle to determine if it is bending or inserting, but the skilled needle therapist will develop a tactile awareness in order to gauge the force necessary to insert.

This is rooted in the idea of "guide, don't push." Most needling pain arises because the practitioner is "pushing"—trying to force the needle through the tissue. This is not necessary, and it will cause resistance and unpleasant sensations for the patient. Instead, the provider must be aware of the tissue and its elasticity, working with the body and moving at its pace. The needle will begin to feel as if it is being drawn into the body, or even moving of its own volition, and the practitioner is merely guiding it to a location and depth. This is the ideal of needle insertion, and is true whether tube or freehand insertion is utilized **(see Video 4)**.

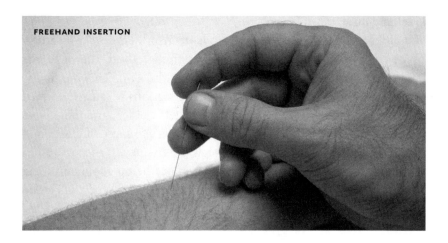

FREEHAND INSERTION

One-Hand Insertion
One-hand insertion is exactly what it sounds like. The needle is held in one hand, whether in a tube or freehand, and inserted without assistance or support of the other hand. This method can be useful in cases where the position of the patient or practitioner makes it difficult to use both hands, or in cases where the other hand is engaged. This could be while supporting a limb in order to access a point, offering pressure at another location for therapeutic purposes, holding an item of clothing out of the way, or for a range of other reasons. This technique is shown in the image above.

Two-Hand Insertion

In a two-hand insertion, the non-needling, or non-dominant hand, will in some way be engaged in the needling process. The most obvious example of this is in tube insertion, where the non-dominant hand will hold the guide tube in place while the dominant hand will tap the needle into the skin. The non-dominant hand can also be used to manipulate the skin in the area of the insertion point. The three most common methods of doing this are stretching, pinching, and pressing.

Stretching is accomplished by using the fingers of the non-dominant hand to pull the skin apart around the point, holding the area tight and flat. This can help with softer tissue, or tissue that has a lot of movement, such as the skin on the abdomen or hip **(see Video 5)**.

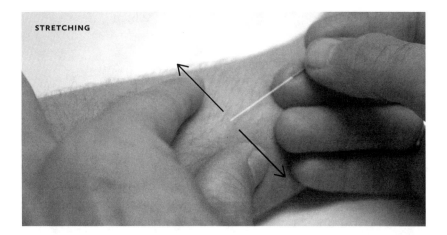

STRETCHING

Pinching is the opposite of stretching. The fingers will be used to draw up tissue to create a block of tissue into which the needle can be inserted. This is useful in places where the skin is tight, or the tissue is shallow and does not allow much space for insertion, such as on the wrists, face, or scalp. This method can also help with oblique and subcutaneous insertions, as it will create a space under the dermis where the needle can pass **(see Video 6)**.

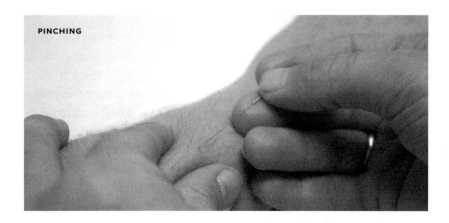

Pressing is accomplished by pressing into the tissue near the point with a finger or thumb of the non-dominant hand. This will serve the dual purpose of stabilizing the tissue, while also reducing the needling sensation for the patient **(see Video 7)**.

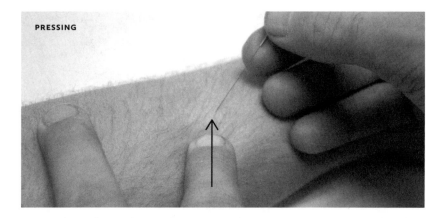

It is important to bear in mind when using a second hand to manipulate tissue during insertion that this manipulation can alter the angle of insertion after it is released. On some occasions, this might not matter to the provider, but in instances where needle angle is being used to manage safety, or where it has been selected to create a specific therapeutic effect, this can be important. With practice, a clinician will become accustomed to accounting for the manipulations of the non-dominant hand, but until that time, a readjustment of the needle might be necessary after initial insertion.

The Non-Dominant Hand

While there are places where a one-hand insertion might be useful, it is important to point out that the non-dominant hand should never be entirely neglected. When we discussed posture previously, it was noted that balance is an important element in creating a strong, comfortable, and effective treatment. Part of the process of creating balance is making sure the engagement is present throughout the body, and this includes the non-dominant hand, even if it is not obviously being used. Whether it is simply laid lightly on the table, held in a ready position, or held actively against the practitioner's own body, it should never be allowed to simply hang passively. There is an idea that appears in some qigong practices, and often in taiji, that if energy is going to be moved in one direction, it must also be moved in the other. In taiji, this can mean the pushing hand opposed by a bracing foot. In needling, this can be the balance between the two hands. If we are to engage deeply and actively with the needling hand, then we must engage the other hand as well.

Regardless of the methods of insertion selected by the provider, there are several basic considerations that should be addressed in any needle insertion. Prior to inserting a needle into a patient, the provider must establish a connection with the patient. This can be accomplished during the intake through good clinical demeanor such as eye contact and interpersonal warmth, but it must be maintained leading up to and during insertion. The patient does not simply become a body and a target for needles once the treatment begins.

Good and mindful physical contact can also help. Active palpation of points will help deepen this connection, maximize location of points, and help mobilize the wei qi (defensive qi) in the desired area so that the body will be less reactive and the insertion less painful.

DEPTH OF INSERTION

Depth is, of course, a major concern in needle treatment. Depth is important for safety, as there are structures underlying the acupuncture cavities in the body that should not be touched or punctured. Depth is also important as it can affect the treatment principles being enacted. For example, external disorders are typically treated at the most superficial depth.

Palpating Acupuncture Cavities

Though this is not a book on point location, it is worth mentioning that the sensitivity of needle insertion and manipulation begins with the palpation of the points. It is a given that the quality of tissue at a point will differ from that around it. Through attention and accurate palpation, the character and nature of the point can be discovered, along with an accurate location, even before the needle is inserted. This can be significant diagnostic information. It will also be of great advantage to the needle therapist when moving the needle through that tissue, and attempting to gain a sense of the deeper structures.

For both these reasons, it is critical for a needle therapist to be able to effectively and actively identify the depths and tissues during the process of needle insertion. A visual understanding of depth can be useful, but overall will prove wholly inadequate to a real mastery of depth, and needling in general. The clinician should strive to develop a personal vocabulary of sensation related to the depth of the needle in the body. As is true with so much of TCM, it is only when we understand what is normal that we can understand what is abnormal, and work to correct it. Just like learning pulses, the needle therapist must feel countless tissues to develop a real fluency in the sensations to be discovered. Once this fluency is present, the insertion of a needle becomes not only therapeutic, but diagnostic, and the feeling of the body's tissues can be used as a guide to the efficacy of manipulation during the treatment process.

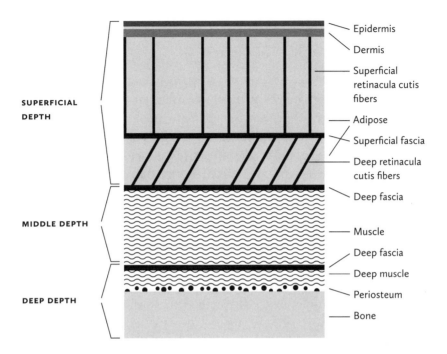

SUPERFICIAL
DEPTH

MIDDLE DEPTH

DEEP DEPTH

— Epidermis

— Dermis

— Superficial
retinacula cutis
fibers

— Adipose

— Superficial fascia

— Deep retinacula
cutis fibers

— Deep fascia

— Muscle

— Deep fascia

— Deep muscle

— Periosteum

— Bone

The depths, like so many things in TCM, are divided into three. These are commonly called superficial, middle, and deep, though different schools of thought will use different terms. What is important here is not the specific terminology but that we understand we are discussing three basic layers of tissue, beginning closest to the skin surface and moving down toward the bone. The transition from layer to layer, if we begin from the outside and move inward, is a process of transition from yang to yin. The exterior of the body and even the wei qi field beyond it are the most yang of all the layers we will touch, with the most changeability, malleability, and movement in the tissue. As we move deeper, we move into more solid structures and active muscles, then deeper into postural muscles, and deeper still into the bone itself, which is predominantly yin in the system of depths. As with all things yin and yang, this is relative and self-relational, with each layer being more yin or yang than the layer below or above it, and all having yin and yang aspects within.

Although there is a variance of tissue throughout the body, there are certain tissue types expected at each one of the depths. By familiarizing ourselves with these tissues and the sensations we can associate with each, we can determine the current depth of the needle by feel alone.

Superficial Depth

The superficial depth begins at the skin surface, or even above it if we take into account the wei qi and our ability to interact with and affect it. Through and interwoven within the wei qi is the epidermis and dermis. At this level, we encounter the initial resistance felt upon needle insertion, and unless great care is taken to keep the needle very shallow, this area will almost always be passed on initial push. Beneath this, we encounter a layer of adipose tissue. This is also a part of the superficial level. The adipose, as opposed to the dermal layer, will feel soft, almost like moving the needle through butter. This layer is certainly not without structure, as the superficial retinacula cutis fibers run through the adipose, connecting the dermis above to the fascia below. When manipulating at this level, it is these fibers that will engage the needle most directly.

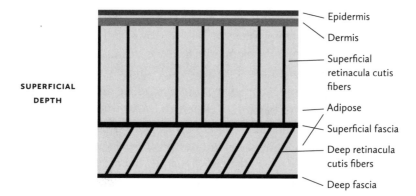

The thickness of this level can vary greatly, depending on where the point being treated is located. Some areas will have thicker skin and a wide adipose layer, such as the lower back, abdomen, and hips, whereas other areas will have very little tissue at this depth, such as the wrists, ankles, or face. It takes a very delicate hand to enter into and remain in the superficial level.

The clinician should also assess the state of the patient's qi at this level through careful sensory exploration. This is the level at which we are in contact with the wei qi, as well as the more superficial channels and luo branches of the 12 meridians.

Middle Depth

The middle depth is comprised principally of the muscle and the fascia that borders it. Like the transition into the superficial depth, the transition to the middle depth is marked by a brief resistance, as the exterior plain of fascia over the surface of the muscle must be pierced. This can be compared to pressing down into a trampoline before it gives way and allows passage into the muscle. The muscle will allow greater movement than pressing through the fascia, but will feel tighter and more structural than the adipose.

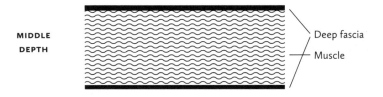

The clinician can gain a powerful view of the patient's systems at this level, as there is contact with both the primary meridian and the very active muscular pathways associated with the channel. This tissue will be very responsive to manipulation, as the practitioner can generate reaction not only from the fascia and its connections, but also in the muscle tissue. The muscles are often the largest structures the practitioner encounters during needle therapy, and are at the level of most needle insertions.

Deep Depth

Beneath the superficial muscle there is another layer of fascia. Depending on the anatomy, this may pass into a deep muscle or straight to bone. Regardless, this is the deep depth. The muscle found here is usually more postural, and composed of denser slow twitch fibers designed for long-term positional holding. Because of this, it will typically feel tighter and slightly harder than the muscle above. Beyond this, or immediately after the first muscular layer, if there are no deeper muscles at a particular location, the clinician will find the periosteum and bone.

Developing Sensitivity

The most effective way to develop sensitivity is through practice on an actual body so that the tissues may be experienced directly. However, it requires thousands of needle insertions to develop the kind of sensitivity needed by a skilled clinician, and there are times when a tissue allegory can be helpful in practice. There are many things that can be put to use. The practitioner can practice insertions on various types of fruit, which will offer not only resistance but also various kinds of "tissue" that can be tested and felt through the needle. Cotton balls can be packed tightly and wrapped in a handkerchief folded several times over, again to simulate skin and the layers beneath. A bar of soap, a book, or even layers of paper tucked between layers of a towel can all offer the dedicated practitioner opportunities to explore insertion and sensation through the needle.

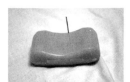 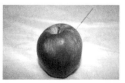 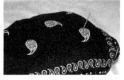

The periosteum is a dense layer of vascular and connective tissue that encases the bone, and although dense, tends to have a spongy quality that can be detected. Bone will have no give at all. If the sponginess extends into the bones, it can indicate a deficiency of the yin, especially of the kidneys.

Many clinicians are hesitant to move the needle near bone, but this concern is unfounded, as it is typically not painful for the patient when you reach the bone, and there is a great deal of stored energy at this depth that can be utilized for the purpose of treatment.

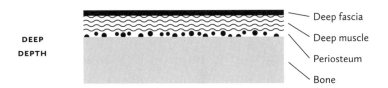

DEEP DEPTH

Deep fascia
Deep muscle
Periosteum
Bone

ANGLE OF INSERTION

The possible angles of insertion are divided into three categories. These are perpendicular, oblique, and transverse (sometimes called subcutaneous). One of the most important considerations is that the angle of insertion is always determined in relation to the skin surface where the needle is being placed. Bear in mind that there are very few flat surfaces on the body, therefore the clinician is not always standing directly in line with the tissue plane, and could be reaching around or across the body to insert a needle.

There are several reasons why controlling the angle of insertion is important. As always, safety comes first. In certain areas of the body, a perpendicular or deep insertion could compromise anatomical structures. This can especially become an issue in areas where nearby clothing could put pressure on an inserted needle, or the patient could move, either of which could cause the needle to move deeper than the original insertion. Inserting the needle at a more shallow angle can prevent the possibility of pushing it inward, as it will move across the line of the body rather than deeper into it.

Angle can also be used to control depth in order to maintain a desired treatment. For instance, if the practitioner wants to treat at a superficial depth with stronger stimulation, it can be advantageous to insert the needle transverse, thereby allowing more needle to be inserted and manipulated without further depth. Conversely, if the clinician wants to reach a deeper depth for treatment, it will require a steeper angle of insertion.

The angle can also be used as a method to direct qi sensation in the patient. We will discuss propagation and globalization of qi sensation in Chapter 5, but for the moment, it is worth stating that the direction of the needle tip can prompt movement of sensation. This same concept can also be used in relation to tonification and sedation, which will also be discussed at length in the same chapter.

Perpendicular

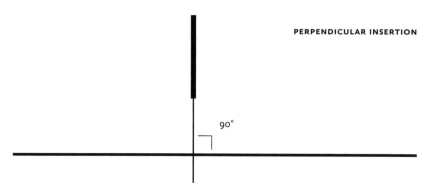

PERPENDICULAR INSERTION

A perpendicular insertion is any insertion where the needle vertically exits the skin at a 90-degree angle with the skin surface. Remember that angle of insertion is related to the surface of the skin, not the position of the clinician.

Oblique

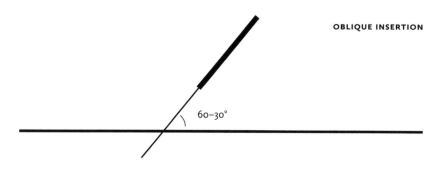

OBLIQUE INSERTION

An oblique insertion is approximately a 60–30-degree angle. The classic angle is 45 degrees, but some variance is reasonable, and is within the judgment of the clinician. This is used to protect deeper structures while still reaching to a middle depth, or in areas of shallower tissue.

Transverse

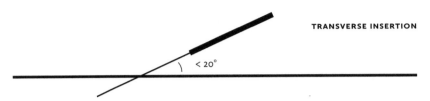

TRANSVERSE INSERTION

< 20°

A transverse insertion is a 20-or-less-degree angle. This insertion is also sometimes called subcutaneous, as the needle typically remains just below the skin surface. This is valuable in areas where there is very little depth of tissue, such as wrists or scalp, as well as maintaining a shallow depth of insertion to present enough needle body within the tissue for dynamic manipulation **(see Video 8)**.

Change of Angle
Occasionally it is necessary to change the initial angle of insertion. This could be due to a desired change in treatment focus, as part of a specific technique, or simply because the angle upon insertion was different than desired. It is unnecessary to completely withdraw the needle and subject the patient to another insertion. Instead, the careful clinician may withdraw most of the needle, bringing it close enough to the skin surface, usually just in the adipose layer, then it will be able to move freely. At this point, the needle can be re-angled and guided back to the desired angle and depth. This technique requires practice and sensitivity, but with a measure of both, is consistently effective.

CULTIVATING SKILLS
At this juncture, the practitioner is prepared to arrange the patient, themselves, and the treatment environment. We have discussed methods of inserting the needle, and how to locate and control both depth and angle. Before moving on, I would encourage a focused practice of these basic skills. Though much of the character of an acupuncture treatment will grow from creation of qi and tonification or sedation, these aspects are built on a solid foundation of the basic practices of insertion, depth, and angle. Without a fluency in these fundamental elements, the

clinician will be stuck having a conversation in idioms, with no real understanding of the vocabulary at their disposal.

The skills discussed in the next chapter are invaluable, but they also require an intense focus all of their own, and to try to learn to execute them without first being comfortable with the previous abilities will only scatter the clinician's focus.

4: DE QI

Once the needle has been inserted, it is necessary to engage the body. To return to the metaphor of a conversation, it is useless to talk to a person if they don't know they are being addressed. You must first get their attention, then wait to be acknowledged. Only then can you commence a dialogue. This moment of attention and acknowledgment is de qi, or the arrival of qi.

De qi has been a topic of some discussion in recent years, with the question arising as to its importance. Studies have found that the presence and strength of de qi sensation in patients had no effect on clinical outcome. Moreover, many patients will experience very little sensation from an acupuncture treatment with even the strongest stimulation, while others will experience significant discomfort with almost no stimulation. As it is often demonstrated, the de qi moment can be quite startling, perhaps even uncomfortable for patients. Patients might experience pressure, numbness, pinching, tingling, warmth, and other sensations.

What is critical to understanding this varied nature of patient response is the nature of de qi. We translate de qi as the arrival of qi, but what does it mean for qi to arrive? As far as channel manipulation and needle therapy are concerned, qi is essentially function, so de qi is the arrival of function, or more specifically, a functional change in the system being contacted. The analogy above continues to serve, as we can imagine de qi to be the turn of a head or nod of the other person to acknowledge that they hear us. In the case of a needle, it is the shift in the sensations of tissue quality felt by the clinician that indicates that the body is now engaged.

What Is Qi?

This is a question that has plagued modern Chinese Medicine. It is a medicine that uses the term qi with such frequency that it is almost defined by it, but at the same time, struggles to define it to the satisfaction of many. This book will not attempt to answer that question, because like so many things in Chinese Medicine, the definition depends on the context. Traditional Chinese is a pictorial language where words represented not sounds alone, but concepts that could be explored, depending on how they were drawn. This leaves a great deal of interpretation to the individual in the situation, and though this can make definition difficult, it is also one of the great strengths of TCM; it exists in context of each treatment. That being said, some general concept of qi is necessary to understand this text, so we will define it as "function." Where Western Medicine is concerned with structure; "what is the heart and what does it do as a structure?"—TCM is more concerned with the relational nature of the body; "how do the heart and the liver interact?" This interaction and functional engagement, which exists finitely in each moment of life, is the core of qi. Therefore, when we talk about qi, we are talking about the body's active response to stimuli, both internal and external.

The other analogy that is often used in relation to de qi is that of someone fishing and feeling their line tugged by a fish beneath the surface. This is certainly a sensation that can be associated with de qi, but it is far from the only one. If the tissue is already hypertonic, then what is there to grasp the needle when de qi is sought? In such a case, the clinician might feel a yielding or softening of the tissues to indicate that the body is responding to the needle and the manipulations. What is really important is that the sensation of de qi is experienced by the practitioner.

Although it has been established that the presence of de qi in the patient has little effect on clinical outcome, the presence of de qi for the clinician is all-important. Though not every patient will experience de qi, it is crucial for the clinician to experience de qi with every patient.

This can be an incredibly subtle sensation, but with practice it is detectable and often can be felt even before a sensitive patient responds to de qi. This is valuable, as it can lessen the discomfort sometimes associated with the arrival of qi. If the practitioner has a sense of de qi before the patient does, the practitioner can control that reaction rather than simply manipulating the needle until the patient jumps.

It is also important to differentiate between the sensation of insertion and de qi. Many patients will feel the insertion, though with skill it will not be painful. This brief passage through tissue, however, is not real engagement but just a passing contact. It is possible that the body will then continue to react and de qi will be achieved upon insertion, but this should never be assumed. The clinician must remain sensitive to and aware of the tissue to ensure full engagement of the body before treatment begins.

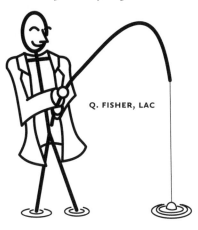

Q. FISHER, LAC

When attempting to attain the de qi sensation—for the patient, and especially for the clinician—there are a number of techniques that can help to stimulate the response. Any of these techniques can be independently used or combined until adequate de qi is attained.

Rotating

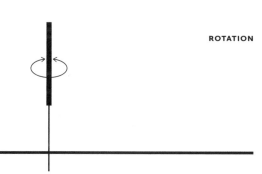

ROTATION

Rotation of the needle is one of the most basic techniques available to the needle therapist. It is touched on at many levels in Chapters 5 and 6 of this book, but for the moment, we must address its use to attain de qi in patients. The method is very simple: the needle is simply rotated in the tissue. The rotation can be large or small, slow or fast, all depending on the overall nature of treatment the clinician desires to create. What should be noted is that although one direction of rotation might be favored, it is best to rotate the needle back and forth. Even the smoothest acupuncture needle will pick up tissue, especially fascia, and one-directional rotation will eventually wind this tissue tightly around the needle. This becomes very uncomfortable for a patient and can lead to stuck needles **(see Video 9)**.

Lifting and Thrusting

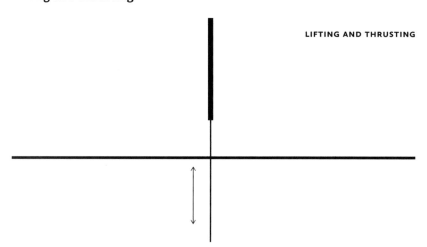

LIFTING AND THRUSTING

In lifting and thrusting, the needle is drawn upward through the tissue and then guided back to depth. The amplitude can be large or small, the motion slow or rapid, though in any technique it is important that the clinician never moves faster than their awareness can keep up with. Before any lifting and thrusting technique is utilized, the needle is guided to the maximum depth of insertion to open up the full breadth of tissue to be stimulated during manipulation, as this will decrease any discomfort experienced by the patient **(see Video 10)**.

Plucking

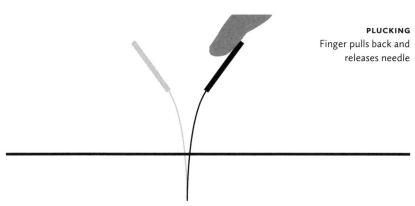

PLUCKING
Finger pulls back and
releases needle

In plucking, the needle is flicked or pulled lightly and released to generate a vibration that will engage the tissues. The amplitude of movement can be large or small, depending on the stimulation desired, though plucking slightly disperses. This can be repeated several times, but in order to determine de qi, it is necessary to return periodically to the handle of the needle and test the response of the tissue between plucks **(see Video 11)**.

Scraping

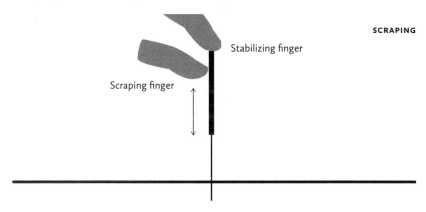

SCRAPING

Stabilizing finger

Scraping finger

Scraping is a method that relies largely on the wire wrapping of the needle handle. This is not to say that it cannot be accomplished on needles that lack the wrapped handles, but wire wrapping makes the process easier. In scraping, the fingernail is dragged up or down the handle, over the wrapping, in order to create a vibration in the needle. Another finger is used to stabilize the needle so that it doesn't move like plucking or shaking but rather focuses on very small and rapid vibrations. The stabilizing finger needs to be above the scraping finger, or the vibrations will be blocked by the lower fingers. As with plucking, it is important to return to the needle regularly to determine tissue response (**see Video 12**).

Shaking

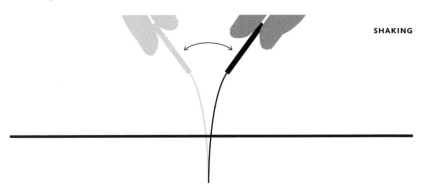

SHAKING

Shaking can be executed in several ways. The needle can be moved back and forth, rotated in a circle, or any other pattern the clinician desires. The core principle of shaking is grasping the needle handle and moving it back and forth, with the point of insertion being the fixed point. This creates a similar needle movement to plucking, but the intensity can be more directly controlled or sustained because the needle is never released (**see Video 13**).

Flying

Flying is a useful technique, not only for acquiring de qi, but also for general stimulation, especially sedation. The technique is executed by lightly rotating the needle back and forth between the fingers and then "flying" the fingers off the needle with a strong final rotation. It is important in this technique that the fingers are not simply lifted off the needle, but that they strongly rotate the needle as they are pulled away.

What this does is engage the body with the initial light rotation, then gives one strong burst of stimulation once that energy is gathered. This can vigorously bring qi to the area, and also help to disperse local stagnation **(see Video 14)**.

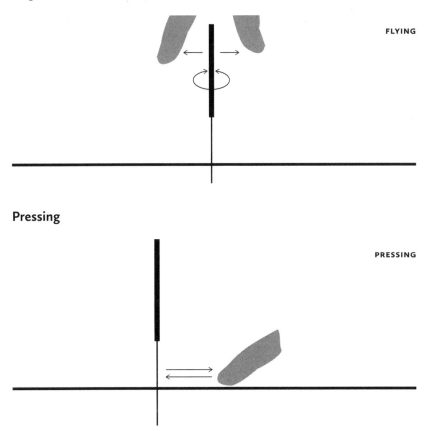

FLYING

Pressing

PRESSING

Not all needle techniques have to directly involve the needle. In pressing, the importance of the non-dominant hand is emphasized by its use to tap, press, or massage the channel where the needle has been inserted. This is done in order to increase stimulation and tissue response to the presence of the needle. This technique can be especially useful when the clinician is having a difficult time achieving de qi with other methods of needle stimulation **(see Video 15)**.

SELECTION OF TECHNIQUE

Each of these techniques can help engage the patient's tissue with the needle and prepare the body for treatment. It is at the discretion of the clinician as to which technique, or combination of techniques, to use in order to elicit an effect. The response of the tissues should be the ultimate guide, but the ability to recognize and capitalize on these methods comes only with extensive practice.

5: CONTINUATION OF NEEDLE SENSATION

The acquisition of de qi is not the end of the clinician's work—on the contrary, it is only the beginning. Once qi and the functional response it represents is attained, it must be guided and given a treatment principle in order to truly effect therapy. There are two primary components to this process, which we will discuss separately for the purpose of clarity, yet they cannot be separated in actual clinical practice. These are the propagation of needle sensation through the body, and tonification or sedation.

Note on Terminology

It seems impossible to write a text on Chinese Medicine, especially one in English, and not at some point have to address the issue of terminology. This is due to the long history of Chinese Medicine, which is complicated by the vagaries of translation. Often a principle will have several possible terms associated with it, such as sedation versus reduction, excess and deficiency versus repletion and vacuity. What is important in these instances is clarity within the specific text on the part of the writer, and understanding of the general concepts by the reader. I will strive to be consistent in word use, as well as clear in my explanation of the underlying concept I am describing, should you encounter a word that could possibly lead you to a different conclusion.

PROPAGATION OF NEEDLE SENSATION

When we discuss propagation of needle sensation, what we are essentially describing is the functional engagement of body tissues and systems from the site of needle insertion to the area of treatment. Oftentimes a needle cannot be inserted directly into the area in need of treatment. The most obvious example of this would be the treatment of internal disorder. If a patient is suffering from large intestine stagnation, leading to decreased peristalsis and constipation, we cannot put a needle in the actual large intestinal organ. The same is true of treating any internal organ disorder, and can even be true in the case of certain orthopedics. Though we can often treat locally for pain patterns, sometimes it is neither possible nor desirable to do so.

As we cannot always directly treat at the location of the disorder, it is a crucial skill to be able to connect from the site of insertion to the site of treatment to maximize results. The progress of this can be tracked in several ways. One, of course, is by patient response, either via their sensation of the treatment itself, or in shifts of pathological symptoms, such as a decrease in pain. Another method is through the clinician's own sensitivity and awareness of the systems they are affecting.

This skill of indirect connection can be one of the most difficult for the needle therapist to develop, due to our tendency to "feel with our eyes," which is to say that we rely heavily on physical sight to make tactile connections, judgments, and decisions, and it is difficult for us to "connect the dots" below the surface. One thing that can help overcome this challenge is a good theoretical understanding of what we are trying to accomplish. To illustrate this, let us consider a room full of people connected by a string. If the clinician were holding one end of the string, and it was strung through each individual in the room before reaching the person at the other end, it would be possible for the clinician to tug on the string to create a sensation of tugging for that person. The clinician would sense the rigidity of the final person, and perhaps even tension in others along the way.

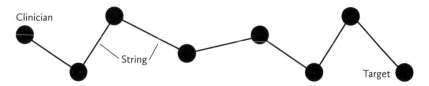

This is the same process that is engaged when needling the channels. We know with immutable certainty that the body is a completely interconnected system, from the epidermis, to the fascia that runs throughout the system, to the blood vessels, nerves, and bones. You cannot affect any one part of it without affecting the whole. The desire is to gain a sensitivity to those effects so that you can actively determine the broader reaction you are creating. There is a simple exercise that a clinician can undertake to aid in developing this skill set.

The most direct approach is to insert a needle at a distal point on a channel. Connect to the local tissue and attain de qi. From there, with the non-dominant hand, press a point farther up the channel, but not across a joint. Maintain contact with the needle, manipulate it, and try to feel the pressure of the non-dominant hand through the tissues at the needle site. Once this is accomplished with ease, simply move the pressing finger farther up the channel. At each phase, the goal remains the same: to be able to feel the effect of the pressing finger through the tissues at the needle site.

METHODS TO IMPROVE SENSATION TRAVEL

Although the principal process of globalizing sensation can be accomplished with the basic manipulations of lifting, thrusting, rotation, and keen sensitivity to tissue response, it is not always enough to insert and manipulate a needle to create a transfer of sensation for either the patient or provider. There are several techniques that can assist in this transmission of connection through the body.

Needle Angle

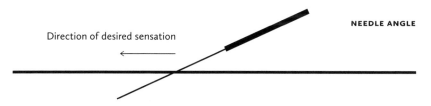

The angle of needle insertion can impact the movement of sensation for the patient. The sensation tends to travel in the direction of insertion. The body experiences the insertion of the needle from the skin surface down, so naturally that sensation will follow the ongoing path of insertion. This means that the needle can be pointed toward the area of desired treatment. If an area is going to be drained or cleared, a distal needle can be inserted away from that point to facilitate movement out of the excess location. A needle could even be inserted in one direction in order to stimulate and make a connection, and then reversed to clear that same area of stagnation or blockage.

Pressing the Needle

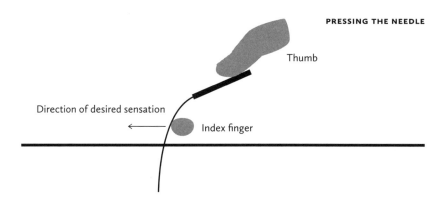

In this method, the index finger and thumb are used to put directional pressure on the needle. This pressure will push the skin slightly in the desired direction, thereby causing a sensation in that same direction. This method can be combined with the angle of the needle, or used on a perpendicular needle, should there be a desire to spread sensation or move in several directions during a treatment without needing to adjust the angle (see Video 16).

Channel Massage/Pressing

Just as in de qi stimulation, pressure on the channel can assist in the creation of sensation. It can physically stimulate the tissue as well as bring the patient's attention to the desired area. In de qi, the channel is usually pressed or rubbed toward the insertion site. Pressing will typically be stimulated in the desired direction of transmission *away* from the needle site. Unlike de qi, where stimulation is usually done in the area of insertion, pressing can be done anywhere along the channel in order to move the sensation onward, across joints, or even from one limb to another **(see Video 15)**.

Joints in Needle Sensation

It has been suggested that the conduction of qi sensation is blocked at major joints. This makes sense, as joints are areas of connection, origin, and termination, where the interconnected tissues a clinician is manipulating are often fixed to solid structures. This also explains why, so often, major acupuncture cavities can be found in the area of joints, as those points would be able to more readily generate effect in both directions from the needled joint. This certainly does not mean that treatments cannot be conducted across joints, thereby requiring only local treatments. Certainly there are very powerful and effective points across the body that are often advantageous to treatment, and a skillful practitioner can easily overcome the issue of transmission across joints. One method that is sometimes employed is to insert a needle in the channel at each joint segment to carry on the treatment response. Alternatively, the pressing method described above can be employed in place of needles to assure connection throughout the system.

TONIFICATION AND SEDATION

Tonification and sedation are a natural extension of globalization of sensation. In these processes, we are beginning to affect the larger system of the meridian and its connected structures, organs, and systems. Returning to the example with the string, we are now not only trying to establish a connection with the distant holder at the end, but working to elicit a specific response.

Though there are a variety of techniques in creating tonification or sedation, which we will discuss, it is important to understand the fundamental character of each. Tonification is slow, gentle, and light, with a mild sensation, whereas sedation is strong, fast, and heavy, with a strong sensation.

This difference can be easily understood in terms of nervous system function. When we engage the body gently, we are able to shift the patient into a more parasympathetic nervous system state, whereas strong stimulation will shift the patient into a more sympathetic nervous system state.

The rest and digest state of recovery and rebuilding, which is associated with the parasympathetic system, mirrors the building impulse of a tonification treatment. Conversely the protection and reaction engagement of the sympathetic system correlates to the clearing and resisting functions of a sedation treatment. This is important to the practitioner in that regardless of what techniques are selected, the underlying character of the manipulation must be controlled. Remember that every patient is different, and what is mild stimulation to one patient might be fairly intense to another. Tonification and sedation must be conducted in relation to the patient's response, not an arbitrary measure of "strong stimulation," so the sensitivity of the clinician must always be paramount in needle treatment.

As with de qi engagement, it is important to guide the needle to the full desired depth before beginning any manipulation, as manipulating through previously unengaged tissue can be very uncomfortable for a patient.

Rotation

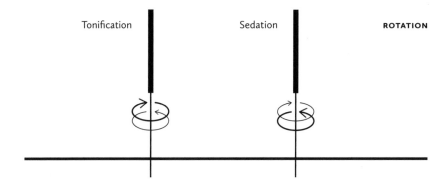

Rotation in tonification and sedation is no different in basic technique than that of de qi stimulation. What is different is an emphasis on one direction of rotation. With tonification, the clockwise rotation will be emphasized, and in sedation, the counter-clockwise rotation will be emphasized. As with de qi stimulation, the needle will still be rotated in both directions for tonification and sedation in order to prevent undesired tissue wrapping on the body of the needle. The direction is an emphasis created by speed of rotation, heaviness of rotation, and intention, rather than repeated twisting in one direction. The emphasized direction will be slightly slower and heavier in technique versus the return twist, which will be light and quick—simply bringing the needle back to the starting position for the next active rotation (**see Video 9**).

To understand this difference, we can consider the anatomical engagement of the needling. The tissue is more likely to pull and move with the needle when the movement is slightly slower and given more emphasis, whereas a light quick movement is more likely to move past the tissue like a table cloth being pulled out from under place settings. When we are selecting a technique for emphasis, the goal is to make sure the tissue is moving with our manipulation in the desired direction.

Lifting and Thrusting

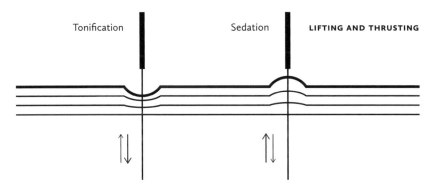

As with rotating, lifting and thrusting is mechanically identical to the method of attaining de qi, save for a directional shift in emphasis. Here, the emphasis for tonification will be on thrusting, and the emphasis for sedation will be on lifting. With tonification, we are building or adding to the body, therefore we emphasize pushing inward. With sedation, we are reducing an excess, and therefore we emphasize pulling outward. As with rotation, emphasis is created by a slower, heavier, more focused movement, with a light movement to return the needle to its starting position for the next lift or thrust.

There is a concrete anatomical reality to this. When we push the needle inward with emphasis (thrust) we are pushing tissues together, compressing and compacting them. This compression will collect and gather blood, lymph, and qi, and thereby increase activity at the point and into the channel. Conversely, when we pull the needle outward (lift), it will pull tissues apart, increasing interstitial space, expanding blood flow, and allowing more movement through the tissue to eliminate points where things have collected, such as stagnations. This is similar to the physical effect of cupping, though far more gentle and localized.

The ideas within lifting and thrusting as a manipulation are present from insertion, all the way to needle withdrawal, with a light quick withdrawal being more tonifying in nature, and a slower, more emphasized withdrawal being more sedating **(see Video 10)**.

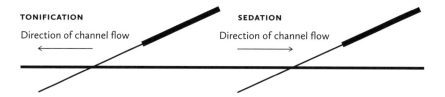

TONIFICATION

Direction of channel flow

←——————

SEDATION

Direction of channel flow

——————→

Needle Angle

We have discussed needle angle as a method of propagating sensation, but it can also be incorporated into the process of tonification and sedation. The simple wisdom is, in needling with the flow of the channel, which is to say the tip of the needle pointing with the flow, you are tonifying, or building. If the tip of the needle points against that flow, then you are sedating, or reducing. This is an easy enough concept to understand as we are either pushing sensation with the channel, which would increase its movement, or against the channel, which would reduce its movement.

The question that must be asked is: "In which direction does a channel flow?" There are several perspectives on this. The most common system used to understand directionality in channel flow is that of the horary cycle (see also the "Time of Treatment" section later in this chapter). Yin channels of the hand flow from the body to the hands, yang channels of the arm flow from the hand to the head, yang channels of the foot flow head to foot, and yin channels of the foot flow from the foot to the body. This flow is relatively easy to remember, as it is mapped by the numbering of the acupuncture cavities. Ascending numbers indicate direction of flow. For example, the lung channel starts in the chest at Lu 1 (Zhongfu) and moves to the hand at Lu 11 (Shaoshang).

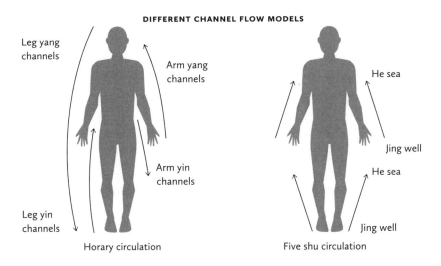

DIFFERENT CHANNEL FLOW MODELS

Leg yang channels

Arm yang channels

He sea

Arm yin channels

Jing well

He sea

Leg yin channels

Jing well

Horary circulation

Five shu circulation

An alternative approach to channel flow can be seen in the nature of the five shu points of each channel, which begin with the jing well points at the fingers and toes, and flow in toward the body and the he sea points at the knees and elbows. In some cases, this will mirror the horary cycle, but can also oppose it. This same extremity inward flow can also be seen in the systems of root and branch, and origin and concentration within the channel systems, all coming together to create a strong alternative to the usually regarded horary flow. With two obviously strong possibilities for channel flow, which direction should be selected in needle angle when tonifying and sedating?

There is no single answer to this question. In fact, it will depend largely on how the channel is being engaged. If a single channel is being used, and if shu points are being selected, then the flow from jing to he points is applicable. However, if the relationship between channels, especially connected channels, is being utilized in treatment, then the horary cycle will be more appropriate. Ideally, the choice will be based on the sensation of the patient and the skilled clinician, that is, not only on intellectual information, but also on direct sensation engagement with the patient's channel response.

Patient Breathing

Breathing can be used to add emphasis during insertion or manipulation, though it is used most commonly with insertion. The focus is on inserting, or manipulating in connection with the patient's inhalation or exhalation. Inserting on the patient's exhalation is considered to be more tonifying in nature, whereas inserting with their inhalation is seen as more reducing. This process can be understood from a qi perspective as a process similar to osmotic pressure. When a patient exhales, the volume of qi in the body will be slightly decreased, creating a gradient that will draw qi in with the insertion. If the patient is inhaling during insertion, then qi is moving into the body via the breath, and it will create an increased internal pressure that will push excess outward, creating a process of sedation.

"OSMOTIC" PRESSURE OF QI WITH BREATH

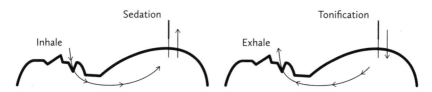

Though this is emphasized during insertion, the same idea can be applied during manipulations, using tonifying techniques during exhalation and sedating techniques during inhalation, and using the opposite breath for the return motion. For example, use a strong clockwise twist with exhalation, and a light return rotation on inhalation.

This process can be understood from the standpoint of physiological function as well. We have already discussed the sympathetic and para-sympathetic nervous systems in relation to tonification and sedation.

These two systems engage with each breath, a process that can most easily be seen in the fact that the heart speeds up slightly with each inhalation and slows slightly with each exhalation, which is known as sinus arrhythmia. This process is controlled by the vagus nerve which is the primary governor of the parasympathetic nervous system. What this means to us is that the body moves slightly toward a parasympathetic state (more tonifying) with each exhalation and into sympathetic (more sedating) with each inhalation.

The clinician can match this breathing pattern during treatment as well. Through careful observation, the practitioner can bring their breath into rhythm with the patient. This will not only help the clinician to be more connected to the patient, but will further emphasize the tonification and sedation aspects of breathing while executing insertions or techniques.

This type of breath control can take a great deal of time to master, and especially to make it a natural part of a treatment environment where so many things are competing for the provider's attention. Its importance cannot be overemphasized, however. Air, and in fact breath, is central to the idea of qi, and a pivotal part of its formation. Regulating the breath is one of the three fundamental regulations of qigong. Even the Chinese character for qi

CHINESE CHARACTER FOR QI

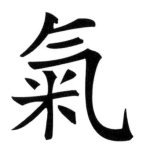

represents a bowl of rice with steam rising from it; an illustration of the combination of food and breath. With breath being so central to the idea of qi, and much of the practice of Chinese Medicine relating to qi, it would be a grave error to neglect the breath of patient or provider in needling practice.

Opening and Closing the Acupuncture Hole
Another concept that arises in terms of tonification and sedation is the ending treatment of the hole made by the acupuncture needle. The idea is that any hole created in the body, and also in the wei field of the body, can allow for the release of some qi. This is why in cases of deficient patients, the number of needles will be reduced. Some styles of practice

will use small needle numbers in all cases, because each needle represents qi lost by the patient. What this means in terms of treatment character— tonification versus sedation—is that if the acupuncture points are left open, or are widened, the treatment will continue to sedate, even after the needle is removed as qi continues to escape from the opened cavity. Conversely, a provider desiring a more tonifying treatment will minimize or close the acupuncture hole.

Needle Withdrawal and Bleeding

There are times where needling will draw blood. It is rarely a significant amount, and almost never dangerous in any way, or requiring more than a few seconds of direct pressure to stop. If there is more severe bleeding, or if the patient has a bleeding condition, an increased duration of pressure will typically prove sufficient. That being said, bleeding at a needle site is not always a negative outcome, nor should it always be addressed immediately. If the desired effect of a point was sedation, especially if the condition was one of a blood or qi stagnation, a few drops of blood can help increase the sedative effects of the treatment. The clinician should observe the bleeding to make sure there is no issue, and then watch the quality of the blood itself. Usually a needle site will offer no more than two or three drops, but the final drop will often change in character from the first, becoming thinner, fresher, and brighter red. At this time, moderate pressure with a cotton ball for 15–30 seconds should be adequate to stop the bleeding.

Closing the acupuncture hole is a simple process, and is typically done simply by pressing the needling site with a finger or cotton ball immediately following withdrawal of the needle. To leave the hole open, the point is not pressed. If a stronger sedation is desired, the needle can be rotated through small or large amplitudes before it is withdrawn, to mechanically increase the size of the hole left by the needle. This can be done with shaking or flying style manipulations.

Needle Order

There are countless methods of tonification and sedation available to the needle therapist—far too many to include in a single book. We will include a few of the lesser-used methods to familiarize the reader with the possibilities, but there are always more to discover. One of these methods relates to the order of needle insertion.

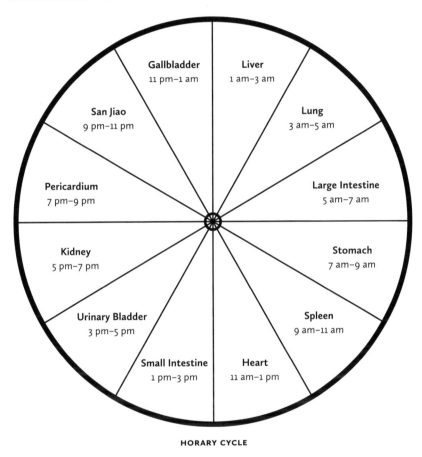

HORARY CYCLE

There is a concept of global qi movement in the body that arises from the five element theory, in which qi naturally flows up the left side of the body and down the right. As in needling with and against the channels, this natural rhythm can be augmented for tonification, or opposed for sedation. This is done, not by needle direction, but by the order of insertion, with treatments that start on the left foot, move up the left side of the body and down the right being seen as more tonifying, while treatments that move in the opposite direction are seen as more sedating in nature.

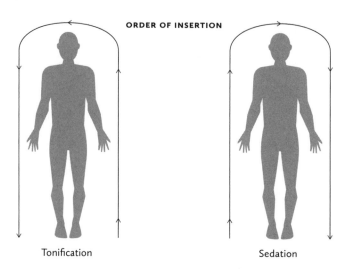

Tonification   Sedation

There are multiple ways to decide on the order of needle insertion, and this is only one of them. What is really of central importance is that the clinician is making an active decision when selecting insertion and withdrawal orders.

Time of Treatment

We have already mentioned the horary flow in relation to channel direction, but it can affect tonification and sedation on another level. The horary flow is connected to the 24 hours of the day in three-hour blocks, with each block being tied to a specific zong or fu organ. The hour associated with the organ is considered the time when that channel and system is most full of qi, and 12 hours opposite, when it will be at its lowest. Through an osmotic gradient process similar to the breath, we can use this to affect tonification and sedation. If treatment is affected during the organ's pertaining hours when it is most full of qi, then the treatment will be more sedating, as the full qi will push pathologies out of the body. Alternatively, if the treatment is given at the 12-hour opposite, then the treatment will be more tonifying, as the lower level of qi will draw qi in from the outside environment.

This method is rarely used, however, because it would require prior knowledge of the patient's pathology to schedule an appointment, and in the case of new patients, or patients with new patterns, this is difficult. In addition, the clinician would have to work on a 24-hour schedule to be able to see patients at the required times. For instance, in a case of lung excess, the practitioner would ideally see the patient between 3 am and 5 am, a time when most providers are not working.

What is more important to draw from the idea of treatment time is that the patient's body is not a static system, and though we might not treat them at the "ideal" time, we can always seek to be aware of their state during any given visit. This will make us more responsive to their constitution in the moment, and allow us to actively engage the channel system during each treatment.

EVEN TECHNIQUES

We have discussed tonification and sedation at length, but it is important to note that not all techniques require one of these two characters. Between the two of them is the possibility of even techniques, which neither tonify nor sedate, but activate, regulate, and move. We will not cover even techniques, as they are the same as the techniques of tonification and sedation, simply without the emphasis. It is perpendicular needle insertion, with emphasis on both the lift and thrust, etc. This sort of attention is often used at locations serving as anchoring points in a treatment. These points are selected because their function aids the treatment strategy, but they are not the chief points. It can also be used in cases of combined excess and deficiency, or areas where the goal is simply movement in a system, with no other change.

Even technique is not "no technique," or an absence of emphasis, but a balance between what would be a tonifying and sedating technique. The tissues must still be deeply engaged to create an active movement.

TECHNIQUE USES IN TREATMENT

The engagement of de qi, the globalization of sensation, tonification, and sedation are all crucial elements that are active parts of an acupuncture treatment. They are not static or set pieces, put in place and then left. Reevaluation and adjustment of the needles and the treatment is always advisable during any needle therapy. Constant assessment of the pulse, as well as the quality of the channel and the acupuncture cavities, will guide the practitioner to the necessary manipulations moment by moment. It would be a mistake to assume that if a needle is inserted with the intention of tonification, that it must only be a tonifying needle. This would be tantamount to beginning a conversation with a particular script in mind, and then following that script regardless of what the other person said or did.

6: COMPOUND AND COMPLEX TECHNIQUES

The approaches to needle technique thus far have all been simple techniques that can each stand on their own. Most treatments, however, involve complex needle manipulation, using techniques that incorporate several of the methods previously discussed. There are a number of established combination techniques for the purpose of tonification, sedation, or even more extensive processes of qi movement and stimulation.

While these combination techniques can be a powerful tool in any needle therapist's arsenal, it would be a mistake simply to take them at face value. When a painter learns to paint, one of their methods is to copy the works of past masters. This is not in order to give them the ability to endlessly recreate the works of those past masters, but to teach them the brush strokes and how to combine them to create an effect. These techniques are much the same for acupuncturists. They can certainly be used as they are, but they are not cast in stone—they are simply a combination of the basic techniques and concepts already discussed: lift and thrust, rotate, depth, angle, etc.

While it is possible to use these techniques simply as they are given, the clinician who does so will miss the richness of sensation and the ability to arrive at spontaneous technique in relation to patient response. Use these techniques, but as you do, strive to understand the various aspects of them, and how they are put together to create a specific effect. First, it is necessary to break them down and look in detail at their simple components, then, after having put countless hours of practice into those simple techniques, the clinician will be ready to explore these more complex processes.

The first three techniques that will be covered in this chapter (Set the Mountain on Fire, Bring Heaven's Coolness, and Midday, Midnight, Mortar-Pounding Pestle) deal specifically with tonification and sedation.

SET THE MOUNTAIN ON FIRE

This is a tonifying technique. It is used to strengthen function, warm, and activate, as the name would imply. It is a combination of lifting and thrusting, rotating, and depths. In order to perform this technique, the needle is inserted to the deepest desired depth and de qi is attained. From here, the needle is withdrawn to the shallowest depth selected for manipulation. The deepest point and shallowest point will demarcate the extent of the treatment. The range between these two points will be divided into thirds.

SET THE MOUNTAIN ON FIRE

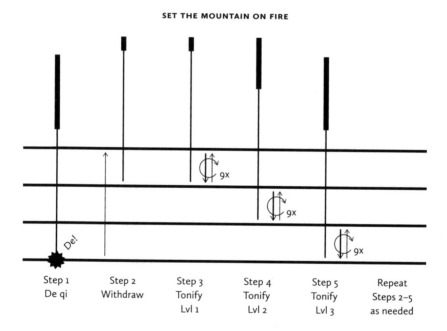

Step 1	Step 2	Step 3	Step 4	Step 5	Repeat
De qi	Withdraw	Tonify	Tonify	Tonify	Steps 2–5
		Lvl 1	Lvl 2	Lvl 3	as needed

Please note: The image of this technique is depicting a single needle in a single acupuncture location, being moved through different depths at different times. It is *not* multiple needles in different locations, *nor* is the needle moved across the tissue during this technique. The label "De!" refers to the arrival of qi.

This space can correspond to the three tissue depths discussed in Chapter 3, or it can be within any one of them, or across two. The range covered will depend on the aspect of the patient in need of tonification. For instance, if the intent is to strengthen the qi and the wei aspect, then the whole of the treatment can be conducted in the superficial depth. Of course, constraining this technique to a single tissue depth will require far greater sensitivity and smaller, finer movements of the needle. When this technique is first learned, it is easier to practice it across the three depths in order to develop a fluidity with the mechanics before trying to compress it into a smaller technique in a single tissue space.

Once de qi is achieved and the needle is withdrawn to the shallowest depth desired, the treatment manipulation begins. The needle will be lifted and thrust, with emphasis on the thrust, while also being rotated, with emphasis on the clockwise rotation. All of this movement will happen in the top third of the divided tissue, and be repeated nine times. Once this is completed, the needle will be moved to the second division and the process repeated. The needle will then be moved to the third depth, and the process of nine times manipulation repeated. Once all these stages have been completed, the needle will be lightly withdrawn back to the shallow depth and the whole process can be repeated again. This can be continued until the desired result is achieved as assessed by pulse, channel palpation, needle sensations, or patient response. At the completion of the technique, the needle is retained at the deepest level. (Typical retention times range from 20 to 30 minutes. For a more in depth discussion of retention times, please see Chapter 7.)

As the name implies, this tonifying technique is warm in character, and if the technique is conducted for long enough, the patient will often feel a sense of strong warmth in the local area, and sometimes even systemically. This can be a desired result, but should be approached with caution in order to avoid overheating the patient (see Video 17).

BRING HEAVEN'S COOLNESS

This is a sedation technique, in contrast to the previous tonification method. This can be used to reduce, cool, sedate, and relax. The basic method is similar to Set the Mountain on Fire in that the tissue is divided into three levels, whether this is the three tissue depths, or three depths within one level. As with any technique, the first step is to take the needle to the deepest desired depth and attain de qi.

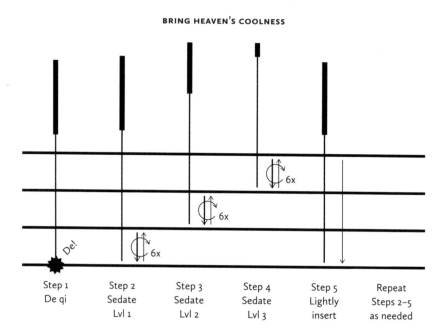

BRING HEAVEN'S COOLNESS

Step 1	Step 2	Step 3	Step 4	Step 5	Repeat
De qi	Sedate	Sedate	Sedate	Lightly	Steps 2–5
	Lvl 1	Lvl 2	Lvl 3	insert	as needed

Please note: The image of this technique is depicting a single needle in a single acupuncture location, being moved through different depths at different times. It is *not* multiple needles in different locations, *nor* is the needle moved across the tissue during this technique. The label "De!" refers to the arrival of qi.

Unlike the previous technique, the needle is not withdrawn to the surface. Instead the technique is initiated from the deepest level. The procedure is essentially the opposite of Set the Mountain on Fire. The needle is lifted and thrust, with the emphasis on the lifting, while also being rotated, with the emphasis on the counter-clockwise direction. This is repeated six times. The needle is then drawn up to the middle level, and the process is repeated, and the process is repeated again at the most superficial level. The needle can then be quickly and lightly thrust back to the deepest level, and the process repeated as many times as is necessary. At the end of manipulation, the needle is retained at the top level **(see Video 18)**. (Typical retention times range from 20 to 30 minutes. For a more in depth discussion of retention times, please see Chapter 7.)

MIDDAY, MIDNIGHT, MORTAR-POUNDING PESTLE

MIDDAY, MIDNIGHT, MORTAR-POUNDING PESTLE

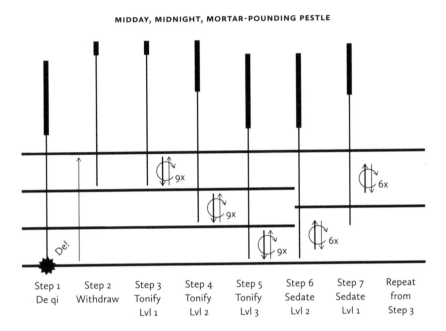

Step 1	Step 2	Step 3	Step 4	Step 5	Step 6	Step 7	Repeat
De qi	Withdraw	Tonify	Tonify	Tonify	Sedate	Sedate	from
		Lvl 1	Lvl 2	Lvl 3	Lvl 2	Lvl 1	Step 3

Please note: The image of this technique is depicting a single needle in a single acupuncture location, being moved through different depths at different times. It is *not* multiple needles in different locations, *nor* is the needle moved across the tissue during this technique. The label "De!" refers to the arrival of qi.

This is a combination technique which brings together the elements of Set the Mountain on Fire and Bring Heaven's Coolness. It is used for patterns of mixed excess and deficiency to be treated at a single point, such as spleen qi deficiency, with dampness treated at Sp 9 (Yinlingquan). Begin by taking the needle to the deepest depth desired and acquiring de qi. From here, you can either begin as you would in Set the Mountain on Fire by withdrawing to the shallow depth of the treatment and then combining tonification techniques down for three levels, or you can remain at the deepest depth and begin treatment from there.

The process is almost exactly the same as it would be for Bring Heaven's Coolness, except the range of treatment is divided into two segments instead of three. Otherwise, the process of six sedating manipulations at each level remains the same.

The choice of whether to start from the deep or the shallow level is based on the clinician's desire to tonify first or sedate. Regardless of where the process is started, the provider will simply alternate between them, tonifying down from the top level and sedating back up from the bottom. This can be repeated for as long as the clinician deems necessary. The needle can then be retained at the surface to emphasize sedation, or at the deepest level to emphasize tonification (**see Video 19**). (Typical retention times range from 20 to 30 minutes. For a more in depth discussion of retention times, please see Chapter 7.)

The following five techniques (Green Dragon Sways Its Tail, White Tiger Shakes Its Head, Green Turtle Burrows the Hole, Red Phoenix Flying, Surrounding Technique) continue to encompass the basic techniques already encountered. They are simply new ways to combine them, but here the manipulation moves beyond simple tonification and sedation, and begins to explore more complex concepts of qi movement and body engagement.

GREEN DRAGON SWAYS ITS TAIL

The green dragon is associated by color and animal with the wood and liver system. The liver, as we know, is tasked with maintaining the smooth flow of qi, and this technique maximizes this effect. It is a combination of needle angle and shaking techniques, and can be used to help direct stimulation down a channel, or to increase flow through an area to break up stagnation and blockage.

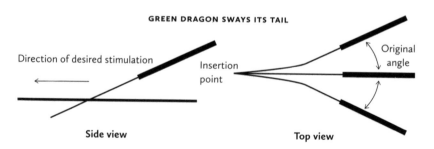

GREEN DRAGON SWAYS ITS TAIL

Direction of desired stimulation

Insertion point

Original angle

Side view

Top view

To perform this technique, the needle is inserted at an angle from oblique to transverse and taken to the desired depth. De qi is attained. Once this is done, the handle of the needle will be shaken back and forth, parallel to the skin surface. Imagine that it is the tail of a dragon or other serpent that is trying to swim up a river, and it is swaying back and forth to push that creature forward. The technique will push qi along the channel in the direction of the needle tip. In cases where the globalization of needle effect is challenging—for instance, if there is stagnation in the channel preventing transmission of sensation—this technique can help move qi through the area. As in any technique, it is important for the clinician to remain connected to the needle and be aware of the patient's response **(see Video 20)**.

WHITE TIGER SHAKES ITS HEAD

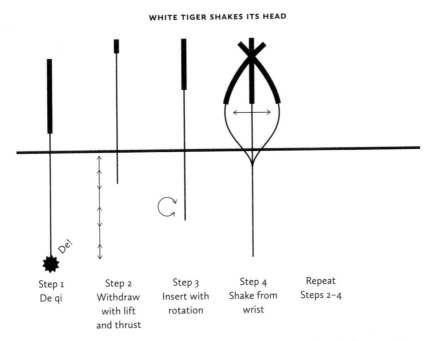

WHITE TIGER SHAKES ITS HEAD

Step 1	Step 2	Step 3	Step 4	Repeat
De qi	Withdraw with lift and thrust	Insert with rotation	Shake from wrist	Steps 2–4

Please note: The image of this technique is depicting a single needle in a single acupuncture location, being moved through different depths at different times. It is *not* multiple needles in different locations, *nor* is the needle moved across the tissue during this technique. The label "De!" refers to the arrival of qi.

White Tiger Shakes Its Head is similar to Green Dragon Sways Its Tail in that it uses shaking to activate its function. However, there are several key differences. Where Green Dragon focuses on the wood action of movement, White Tiger (named after the color and animal of the metal element) embraces the lung's function of dispersing and descending.

The needle is inserted perpendicularly to the full depth of treatment and de qi is acquired. The needle is then withdrawn with light, quick lifting and thrusting and returned to the depth with light rotating. This is repeated several times until the clinician feels that the patient's qi is well engaged with the needle. The needle is then shaken, but this shaking is not the same motion as in Green Dragon. Instead of the needle swaying from the point of insertion, the hand is moved back and forth from the wrist like the head of a tiger shaking prey in its mouth. This has a dispersing effect, expanding the qi out from the point of insertion. This can be repeated until the clinician is satisfied with the result. Often it will create a sense of opening to the patient, and the clinician should be able to feel hypertonic tissue releasing and softening during this process (**see Video 21**). On completion of the technique, the needle can be withdrawn or retained, depending on the overall treatment plan.

GREEN TURTLE BURROWS THE HOLE

This is another technique for spreading and evening out qi. The turtle is an animal of the water element, and the nature of water is to spread and fill, creating evenness from an uneven landscape. Green Turtle can be used to disperse and scatter stuck or stagnant energy, typically from a central point.

The needle is inserted obliquely and de qi is attained using any method the clinician favors. Once de qi is acquired, the needle is withdrawn without actually removing it. The needle is re-angled in the opposite direction and inserted back to depth. De qi is then attained again. The process is repeated two more times at the perpendicular angles. If the clinician desires, the needle can be inserted from additional angles, or the original process can be repeated. (Although Turtle Burrows the Hole is typically done at four different angles, it can be done from as

few as two angles or as many as the practitioner prefers. **See Video 22.**)
On completion of the technique, the needle can be withdrawn or
retained, depending on the overall treatment plan.

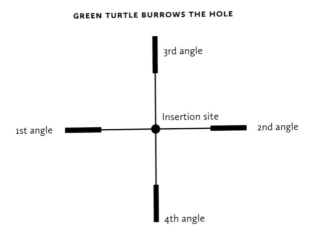

GREEN TURTLE BURROWS THE HOLE

RED PHOENIX FLYING

This is a vigorous and activating technique that mirrors the rising and
warming qualities of the red phoenix (the animal of fire, after which it
is named). To perform this technique, the needle is inserted deeply and
stimulated to de qi. Once this engagement is gained, the needle is lifted
up close to the surface, drawing the qi with it. The needle is thrust slightly
down, and then the flying technique is executed. This is the same flying
technique discussed in Chapter 4. This full process can be repeated until
the desired effect is achieved. Often this technique will create a sense
of spreading warmth or pressure in the area as the powerful energy of
the deeper tissue is drawn upward, and then expanded into the surface
tissues by the flying technique **(see Video 23).**

RED PHOENIX FLYING

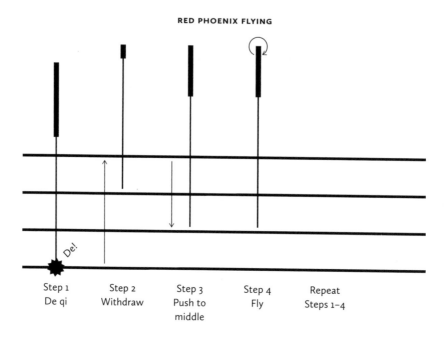

Step 1
De qi

Step 2
Withdraw

Step 3
Push to middle

Step 4
Fly

Repeat
Steps 1–4

Please note: The image of this technique is depicting a single needle in a single acupuncture location, being moved through different depths at different times. It is *not* multiple needles in different locations, *nor* is the needle moved across the tissue during this technique. The label "De!" refers to the arrival of qi.

SURROUNDING TECHNIQUE

Unlike the techniques we have discussed up to this point, the Surrounding Technique uses multiple needles. This technique is very much as it sounds. Multiple needles (two or more) are inserted around a selected area. Although a specific number is not critical to this technique, it is usually done in a balanced fashion, with needles complementing each other from opposing sides of the treatment area. The needles can be inserted pointing toward the desired location to move stimulation into the area, or pointed away from it to disperse energy. The distance between the needles is also under the control of the clinician. A single point can be surrounded for a fixed issue, or the needles can be put further apart in instances of pathology with large muscle groups or broader channel function. With each needle inserted, it is important to attain de qi. Once all the needles are inserted, any additional techniques can be applied in order to create the desired effect of the treatment (**see Video 24**).

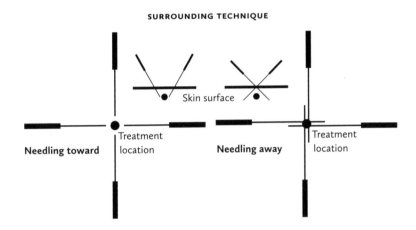

SURROUNDING TECHNIQUE

Skin surface

Needling toward · Treatment location · Needling away · Treatment location

7: DURATION OF TREATMENT, RETENTION OF NEEDLES, AND THE TREATMENT EXPERIENCE

There are as many different versions of an acupuncture treatment as there are acupuncturists. It is not within the scope of this book to define a treatment in absolute terms, so this chapter will be brief and touch on some of the main points in composing overall treatment processes, which have already been covered. This will simply be a place to bring them together.

The most central thing to an acupuncture treatment is the clinician's judgment. In an ideal treatment, everything that happens from the moment the patient sets foot through the front door of the office happens with design and intent. Anyone who imagines the treatment beginning with the insertion of the needle and ending with its withdrawal dramatically misunderstands the space occupied by the clinician, and ignores much of what TCM would teach about holistic therapy. It is impossible to separate the patient's experience from the environment, the clinician, and the treatment. That being said, this is not a book on Feng Shui or personal communication, so we will move forward to the needling portion of the treatment process, having clarified that the events leading up to treatment can have a significant impact upon success.

Probably the simplest way to discuss the process of needle therapy is a simple flow chart of the events in a typical treatment. This will vary, but can establish a general framework that the clinician can consider as they move through the process of treatment. Bear in mind that this list is not mandatory, and that not every step might be used in every case, though just because something isn't done shouldn't mean it isn't considered. The choice to omit something from treatment should be as significant and mindfully done as the choice to include something. At each step, the clinician should strive to control the composition and nature of the treatment.

The Process of Treatment (Following Intake and Diagnosis)
Pre-needling therapies (e.g. cupping, guasha, tuina, etc.)
Point selection
Patient positioning
    Patient safety and comfort
    Needle access
    Provider position
Order of insertion determined
First needle
    Palpate point for location and to engage wei qi
    Determine desired needle angle
        Safety concerns in area
        Depth of local tissue
        Direction of treatment target location
        Tonification and sedation
    Watch and mirror the patient's breath
        Determine desired breath cycle for insertion
    Insert needle with preferred method
    Guide to selected depth
        Safety concerns in area
        Ideal depth for treatment protocol
        Patient's response
    Attain de qi
        Determine initial sensations of current tissue state
        Supply desired stimulation method
        Wait for tissue response
    Globalize sensation
        Connect needling site to desired treatment target

Feel for systemic body connections

Observe patient response

Implement treatment protocol

Tonification, sedation, or even techniques as desired

Reassess pulse, tissue, channel sensation to adjust manipulations

Continue manipulations until desired result is attained

Subsequent needles

Repeat full process from the first needle

Readdress needles

If desired the patient can be reassessed during treatment

Needles can be further manipulated, removed, added to, or replaced

This can be done any number of times throughout the treatment

The clinician may leave the room and return for this or remain and constantly monitor progress

Additional techniques

Moxa, cupping, etc. can be included during the course of needle treatment if desired

Removal

Patient's state is reassessed

Removal order is determined

Removal of first needle

Tissue is tested for final assessment

Final manipulations are conducted

Watch and mirror patient's breath cycle

Needle is removed on selected breath cycle (remove quickly or slowly depending on desired after-treatment effect)

Open or close acupuncture hole as desired

Removal of subsequent needles

Repeat full process from first needle

Additional techniques

Moxa, cupping, etc. can be included after needles are removed if desired

Final patient assessment

After all treatment is completed, conduct final assessment of patient (pulse, tongue, channel palpation, etc.)

This list is neither comprehensive, nor absolute. Variations can arise in even this simple order of treatment, and like a great conductor leading an orchestra, the needle therapist must always be ready to improvise and guide the treatment in a new direction, based on the needs of the patient in that moment. Many techniques, which have arisen over the long and rich history of acupuncture as a practice, are not covered in this list or this text. This book is simply about the most basic practices with a needle, and comprehension can build a solid base to develop further specialized methods.

As to the duration of treatment, there are a wide variety of opinions. Thirty minutes of needle retention is a general average, but there are no hard-and-fast rules. Ultimately, this choice must come down to the clinician's sense about the patient's needs. Sometimes the needle will be briefly manipulated, the body will respond, and the treatment is completed. Other times the body will need to rest with the needle for an hour or more to elicit a response. Bear in mind that retention of needles and duration of treatment is not necessarily the same thing.

When the needles are removed, it often signals the end of the treatment, but this is a time when additional methods such as moxa or cupping may be employed. Perhaps the patient needs to remain on the table to rest and finish absorbing the effects of the treatment. Even after the patient gets up from the treatment table, the treatment can continue with education or guided exercises. The treatment process ends when the patient departs the office.

CLOSING THOUGHTS

This text has not covered a wide breadth of material. Instead, the goal has been to look in more depth than is normally the case at some of the most basic skills of the needle therapist. Although these skills are simple, they are not necessarily easy. The insertion and manipulation of a needle is so central to the practice of acupuncture that it is often neglected as a matter of course. Every acupuncturist can put in a needle, and all of them can manipulate it, but the question remains, "How many have truly cultivated that aspect of their practice?"

Chen Man Ching once suggested that if an individual wanted to develop a skill in calligraphy, it was necessary to draw 10,000 vertical lines before any attempt was made to draw a character. His idea was that, although it seems easy to draw a vertical stroke, this is a misunderstanding—few people can consistently do so because they see it as too basic, and therefore do not practice it enough. These foundational skills are the vertical strokes of our practice.

It is not necessary to follow my needling method, but I hope that this encourages practitioners, old and new alike, to renew an interest in the deeper development of these core clinical skills. Medicine is a practice, and practice we must.

Glossary

Adipose Fat tissue.

Cun A traditional measurement of length. Classically considered to be the width of a person's thumb knuckle.

De qi The response of the body to the techniques of the practitioner.

Dermis The skin.

E-stim A type of acupuncture practice in which electrodes are attached to the needles and a mild current is run through the body tissue.

Epidermis The most superficial layer of the skin.

Fascia A thin sheet or band of fiberous connective tissue that separates and connects various body structures.

Filiform needle A thin, solid (as opposed to hollow) needle which is used in the practice of acupuncture. Filiform means thread-like and describes the small size of modern needles.

Guide tube A plastic tube designed to aid in needle insertion.

Handle The part of the filiform needle held by the practitioner.

Hematoma A bruise.

Horary cycle A circadian cycle of energy flow through the body that highlights the qi focus in certain channels at certain times of day.

Luo branches A secondary set of channels that serve a function of connection through the body.

Martial horse stance A position seen in classic martial arts where the practitioner stands with feet two shoulder widths apart and knees deeply bent.

Meridians The classic energetic and functional pathways of Traditional Chinese Medicine.

Parasympathetic nervous system The rest and digest nervous system, responsible for relaxed body states.

Periosteum The superficial coating of the bone.

Peristalsis The wave-like contractions of the digestive system that assist in the transport of food and waste matter through the body.

Pneumothorax A dangerous medical condition in which air is allowed to leak into the chest cavity, causing the lungs to compress.

Prone Face down.

Qi Functional energy of the body, used to facilitate healing in acupuncture.

Qigong The practice of cultivating internal energy through meditation, breath, and movement.

Retinacula cutis fibers Thread-like fibers that connect the deep dermis to the fascial layers beneath and control skin elasticity and mobility.

Root The point where the shaft of the filiform needle connects to the handle.

Sedation Using techniques to clear blockage, or dissipate excess energy in the body.

Shaft The part of the filiform needle which will be inserted into the body.

Shu points A set of five points on the limbs that create a description of flow from the fingers toward the body, each with specific classical indications.

Sinus arrhythmia A normal change in heart rate during different phases of respiration.

Supine Face up.

Sympathetic nervous system The fight-or-flight nervous system, responsible for heightened body states during a stress response.

Syncope Fainting.

Taiji A traditional martial art that emphasizes soft, relaxed movement and the breath.

Tail A loop on the end of the handle of the filiform needle. Many modern needles no longer have a tail.

Tip The sharp end of the filiform needle.

Tonification Using techniques to increase the functional response of the body.

Wei qi Defensive qi. A layer of active energy that runs around the surface of the body and acts to resist negative outside influence.

Yang The active form of energy, related to warmth, rising, brightness, and movement.

Yin The passive form of energy, related to cool, sinking, darkness, stability, and nourishment.

Index